CONQUERING COLORECTAL CANCER

Your Guide to Understanding, Overcoming, and Thriving

RICHARD BACHMAN

TABLE OF CONTENT

INTRODUCTION TO COLORECTAL CANCER

UNDERSTANDING THE BASICS

Colorectal cancer, a formidable adversary in the realm of oncology, stands as one of the leading causes of cancer-related morbidity and mortality worldwide. In this discourse, we embark upon a journey of enlightenment, delving deep into the intricate tapestry of colorectal cancer, from its humble beginnings to its devastating consequences. With each word penned, we seek to illuminate the path towards understanding the fundamental aspects of this disease, equipping you, the reader, with the knowledge needed to navigate its complexities and challenges.

Understanding the Basics:

Colorectal cancer, often referred to as bowel cancer or colon cancer, arises from the uncontrolled growth of abnormal cells in the colon or rectum, the two components of the large intestine. To comprehend the nuances of this disease, it is imperative to grasp the anatomy and function of these vital organs.

The colon, also known as the large bowel, plays a crucial role in the digestion and absorption of nutrients. It consists of several segments, including the ascending colon, transverse colon, descending colon, and sigmoid colon, each with distinct functions in the digestive process. Adjacent to the colon lies the rectum, a short, muscular tube responsible for the storage and expulsion of fecal matter from the body.

The development of colorectal cancer typically follows a sequence of precancerous changes known as adenoma-carcinoma progression. Initially, benign growths called polyps form on the inner lining of the colon, or rectum. Over time, a subset of these polyps may undergo malignant transformation, giving rise to colorectal cancer.

Risk Factors and Epidemiology:

Colorectal cancer does not discriminate; it affects individuals of all ages, genders, and ethnicities. However, certain factors predispose individuals to an increased risk of developing this disease. Age is a significant determinant, with the majority of cases diagnosed in individuals over the age of 50. Additionally, a family history of colorectal cancer or inherited genetic syndromes, such as Lynch syndrome and familial adenomatous polyposis (FAP), heightens the risk of disease occurrence.

Lifestyle factors also play a pivotal role in the etiology of colorectal cancer. Sedentary behavior, a diet high in red and processed meats, low fiber intake, obesity, and tobacco use have all been implicated as modifiable risk factors associated with the development of this malignancy. Furthermore, conditions such as inflammatory bowel disease (IBD), including ulcerative colitis and Crohn's disease, predispose individuals to an increased risk of colorectal cancer over time.

Symptoms and Early Detection:

Colorectal cancer often progresses silently in its early stages, manifesting minimal or nonspecific symptoms. However, as the disease advances, certain warning signs may emerge, serving as red flags for further investigation. These symptoms may include:

- Persistent changes in bowel habits, such as diarrhea, constipation, or narrowing of the stool
- Rectal bleeding or blood in the stool
- Abdominal discomfort, cramping, or bloating
- Unexplained weight loss or fatigue
- Feeling of incomplete bowel emptying

Early detection of colorectal cancer is paramount to improving patient outcomes and prognosis. Screening tests, such as colonoscopy, fecal occult blood testing (FOBT), fecal immunochemical testing (FIT), and sigmoidoscopy, aim to identify precancerous lesions or early-stage tumors before they progress to advanced disease. National guidelines recommend regular screening for individuals at average risk beginning at age 50, with earlier initiation and more frequent surveillance for those with heightened risk factors.

Diagnosis and Staging:

Upon suspicion of colorectal cancer based on clinical presentation or screening findings, a comprehensive diagnostic workup is initiated to confirm the diagnosis and assess the extent of disease spread. Diagnostic modalities may include:

- **Colonoscopy:** A visual examination of the entire colon and rectum using a flexible, lighted tube equipped with a camera.
- **Biopsy:** removal of tissue samples from suspicious lesions for histopathological analysis to determine the presence of cancer cells.
- **Imaging Studies:** Computed tomography (CT) scans, magnetic resonance imaging (MRI), and positron emission tomography (PET) scans may be utilized to evaluate the

extent of tumor involvement and detect metastatic spread to distant organs.

Following confirmation of colorectal cancer, staging is performed to stratify patients into different prognostic categories based on the size and extent of the primary tumor, involvement of regional lymph nodes, and presence of distant metastases. The TNM staging system, developed by the American Joint Committee on Cancer (AJCC), serves as the standard classification system used for staging colorectal cancer. Staging facilitates treatment planning and prognostication, guiding therapeutic decisions and informing patients about their disease prognosis.

Conclusion:

In the realm of oncology, knowledge serves as a potent weapon in the battle against cancer. Armed with a comprehensive understanding of the basics of colorectal cancer, from its anatomical origins to its diagnostic intricacies, we embark upon a journey of enlightenment and empowerment. As we navigate the complex terrain of this disease, let us remain steadfast in our commitment to unraveling its mysteries, advocating for early detection, and advancing innovative therapies to improve patient outcomes. Together, we stand united in our quest to conquer colorectal cancer and usher in a future free from its grip.

IMPORTANCE OF EARLY DETECTION

Before delving into the significance of early detection, it is paramount to grasp the fundamentals of colorectal cancer. CRC originates in the colon or rectum, typically developing from benign growths called polyps. Over time, these polyps can transform into cancerous lesions, posing a grave threat to health and well-being. Factors such as age, family history, lifestyle choices, and underlying medical conditions can influence one's susceptibility to CRC.

The silent progression of CRC often renders it asymptomatic in its early stages, making detection challenging without proactive screening measures. As the disease advances, symptoms such as rectal bleeding, changes in bowel habits, abdominal pain, and unexplained weight loss may manifest. However, by this stage, CRC may have already reached an advanced state, limiting treatment options and diminishing the prognosis.

Importance of Early Detection:

Early detection serves as a cornerstone in the fight against colorectal cancer, offering a pivotal opportunity for timely intervention and improved outcomes. The significance of early detection is multifaceted, encompassing several key aspects that underscore its critical importance:

1. **Enhanced Treatment Efficacy:** Early-stage colorectal cancer is more amenable to treatment, with higher rates of successful intervention and an improved prognosis. Surgical resection, chemotherapy, radiation therapy, and targeted therapies are among the treatment modalities employed in the management of early-stage CRC. By detecting the disease in its incipient stages,

clinicians can implement appropriate treatment strategies aimed at achieving optimal outcomes and preserving quality of life.

2. **Reduced Mortality Rates:** Early detection of colorectal cancer has been associated with reduced mortality rates, underscoring its potential to save lives. Screening programs aimed at identifying CRC in its early stages have demonstrated significant reductions in mortality, highlighting the efficacy of proactive detection efforts. Through routine screening and timely diagnosis, individuals can mitigate the risk of disease progression and mortality associated with advanced colorectal cancer.

3. **Minimized Disease Burden:** Early detection not only improves treatment outcomes but also minimizes the physical, emotional, and financial burden imposed by advanced colorectal cancer. By identifying the disease at an early stage, patients may avoid the need for extensive surgical procedures, aggressive chemotherapy regimens, and prolonged

hospitalizations. Furthermore, early detection affords individuals the opportunity to preserve normal bowel function and avoid complications associated with advanced CRC, enhancing their overall quality of life.

4. **Cost-Effectiveness:** From a healthcare perspective, early detection of colorectal cancer offers substantial cost savings by averting the need for expensive and intensive treatments associated with advanced disease. Screening programs aimed at early detection are cost-effective investments, yielding long-term benefits in terms of reduced healthcare expenditures and improved productivity. By allocating resources to proactive screening initiatives, healthcare systems can achieve significant returns on investment while promoting population health.

Conclusion:

In conclusion, the importance of early detection in the context of colorectal cancer cannot be overstated. By recognizing the significance of timely intervention, individuals can take proactive steps to safeguard their health and well-being. Screening programs, diagnostic tests, and awareness campaigns play a pivotal role in facilitating early detection and improving outcomes for individuals at risk of colorectal cancer. As advocates for health and wellness, it is incumbent upon healthcare providers, policymakers, and community stakeholders to prioritize early detection initiatives and empower individuals to take charge of their colorectal health. Together, through concerted efforts and unwavering dedication, we can navigate the terrain of colorectal cancer with resilience, determination, and hope.

OVERVIEW OF COLORECTAL CANCER STATISTICS

Colorectal cancer transcends geographical boundaries, affecting individuals across continents and cultures. According to recent estimates from the World Health Organization (WHO), colorectal cancer ranks among the most prevalent cancers globally, with an alarming rise in incidence observed in both developed and developing nations. This insidious disease respects neither age nor gender, manifesting in individuals of varying demographics with a propensity that knows no bounds.

Incidence and Mortality Trends

Delving deeper into the realm of statistics, we confront the sobering reality of colorectal cancer's impact on human lives. The incidence of colorectal cancer has exhibited a concerning upward trajectory in recent decades, attributed in part to shifting lifestyle patterns, dietary habits, and aging populations. Despite advancements in early detection and treatment modalities, colorectal cancer remains a leading cause of cancer-related morbidity and mortality worldwide.

Regional Disparities

While colorectal cancer affects populations universally, the burden of this disease is not distributed evenly across the globe. Disparities in healthcare access, socioeconomic status, and cultural norms contribute to divergent patterns of incidence, mortality, and survival rates observed among different regions and demographic groups. Addressing these inequities is essential to achieving equitable outcomes in colorectal cancer prevention, diagnosis, and care on a global scale.

The Role of Screening and Early Detection

Amidst the stark realities of colorectal cancer statistics, there exists a beacon of hope in the form of screening and early detection initiatives. Evidence suggests that timely screening interventions can significantly reduce the incidence of colorectal cancer and improve survival outcomes through the identification and removal of precancerous polyps or early-stage malignancies. Embracing comprehensive screening programs as integral components of healthcare systems is paramount to mitigating the burden of colorectal cancer and saving lives.

Emerging Trends and Prognostic Indicators

As we navigate the landscape of colorectal cancer statistics, it is imperative for remain vigilant to emerging trends and prognostic indicators that shape the trajectory of this disease. From the advent of precision medicine and immunotherapy to the exploration of novel biomarkers and genetic predispositions, ongoing research endeavors hold promise for enhancing our understanding of colorectal cancer and refining therapeutic approaches tailored to individual patients.

Conclusion: A Call to Action

In conclusion, the panorama of colorectal cancer statistics serves as both a stark reminder of the challenges we face and a rallying cry for collective action. By arming ourselves with knowledge, fostering collaboration across disciplines, and advocating for equitable access to care, we can strive towards a future where colorectal cancer ceases to exert its devastating toll on humanity. Let us embark on this journey with resolve and determination, united in our pursuit of a world free from the grip of colorectal cancer.

UNDERSTANDING COLORECTAL CANCER

ANATOMY OF THE COLON AND RECTUM

Colorectal cancer stands as one of the most prevalent malignancies globally, affecting millions of lives each year. Central to comprehending this disease is grasping the intricate anatomy of the colon and rectum, where colorectal cancer typically originates. In this exploration, we will embark on a detailed journey through the anatomy of these vital structures, illuminating their significance in the context of colorectal cancer development.

The Colon: A Crucial Component

The colon, also known as the large intestine, plays a significant role in the digestive process. It comprises several distinct regions, each contributing to the absorption of water and nutrients, as well as the formation and elimination of waste. Beginning with the cecum, located in the lower right abdomen, the colon ascends on the right side as the ascending colon. It then traverses horizontally as the transverse colon before descending on the left side as the descending colon. Finally, it curves inward towards the midline as the sigmoid colon, leading to the rectum.

The Rectum: Gateway to Elimination

The rectum serves as the terminal segment of the large intestine, connecting the colon to the anus. Positioned within the pelvis, its primary function is to store fecal matter until defecation occurs. The rectum is anatomically distinct from the colon and is characterized by its thicker muscular walls and expanded diameter, allowing for the accumulation and expulsion of stool.

Colorectal Cancer: Origins and Development

Colorectal cancer arises from the uncontrolled growth and proliferation of abnormal cells within the colon or rectum. Most colorectal cancers begin as benign growths called polyps, which can gradually progress to malignancy over time.

Understanding the anatomical features of the colon and rectum is crucial to elucidating the mechanisms underlying cancer initiation and progression.

Polyps: Precursors to Cancer

Polyps are aberrant growths that can develop on the inner lining of the colon or rectum. While the majority of polyps are benign, certain types, such as adenomatous polyps, harbor the potential for malignant transformation. Adenomatous polyps, characterized by dysplastic changes in the epithelial cells, represent the primary precursor to colorectal cancer. Over time, these polyps may acquire additional genetic mutations, leading to the development of invasive cancer.

Location Matters: Understanding Disease Patterns

The anatomical location of colorectal cancer within the colon or rectum influences its clinical presentation, prognosis, and treatment approach. Lesions arising in the right colon tend to present with nonspecific symptoms, such as fatigue and anemia, due to their propensity for occult bleeding. In contrast, tumors located in the left colon or rectum often manifest with symptoms such as rectal bleeding, changes in bowel habits, and abdominal pain, facilitating earlier detection and intervention.

Anatomical Considerations in Diagnosis and Treatment

An in-depth understanding of the anatomical landmarks of the colon and rectum is paramount in the diagnosis and management of colorectal cancer. Diagnostic modalities such as colonoscopy, flexible sigmoidoscopy, and imaging studies rely on precise anatomical knowledge to identify suspicious lesions and assess disease extent. Surgical interventions, including colectomy and rectal resection, aim to remove the tumor while preserving adequate intestinal function, necessitating meticulous attention to anatomical detail.

Beyond Anatomy: Embracing Multidisciplinary Care

While anatomical considerations form the foundation of colorectal cancer management, a comprehensive approach encompassing multidisciplinary collaboration is essential. The treatment of colorectal cancer often involves a combination of surgery, chemotherapy, radiation therapy, and targeted therapies, tailored to individual patient characteristics and disease characteristics. Moreover, advancements in precision medicine and immunotherapy continue to revolutionize the landscape of colorectal cancer treatment, underscoring the importance of interdisciplinary synergy in optimizing patient outcomes.

Conclusion: Illuminating the Path Forward

In conclusion, a profound understanding of the anatomy of the colon and rectum is indispensable in unraveling the complexities of colorectal cancer. By elucidating the intricate interplay between anatomical structures, disease mechanisms, and therapeutic interventions, we can forge a path towards improved detection, treatment, and ultimately eradication of this formidable disease. As we navigate this terrain together, let us remain steadfast in our commitment to advancing knowledge, fostering innovation, and empowering those affected by colorectal cancer on their journey towards healing and hope.

WHAT CAUSES COLORECTAL CANCER?

At the heart of understanding colorectal cancer lies the intricate interplay of genetic, environmental, and lifestyle factors. While the exact etiology remains elusive, researchers have identified several key contributors that shape its pathogenesis.

Genetic Predisposition: Unraveling the Genetic Code

A significant subset of colorectal cancer cases can be attributed to inherited genetic mutations that predispose individuals to the disease. Hereditary syndromes such as Lynch syndrome (hereditary nonpolyposis colorectal cancer) and familial adenomatous polyposis (FAP) underscore the critical role of genetics in colorectal cancer susceptibility. Mutations in genes such as APC, KRAS, and TP53 disrupt cellular homeostasis, fueling the transformation of normal colonic epithelial cells into malignant counterparts.

Environmental Exposures: Navigating the Hazards

Beyond genetic predisposition, environmental exposures play a pivotal role in shaping colorectal cancer risk. Dietary factors, including high consumption of red and processed meats, low fiber intake, and inadequate fruit and vegetable consumption, have been implicated in colorectal carcinogenesis. Furthermore, exposure to environmental toxins such as tobacco smoke, alcohol, and industrial pollutants may exacerbate the risk of developing colorectal cancer, highlighting the pervasive influence of the environment on disease susceptibility.

Lifestyle Choices: The Impact of Behavioral Patterns

The modern lifestyle, characterized by sedentary behavior, poor dietary habits, and escalating rates of obesity, has emerged as a significant contributor to the rising incidence of colorectal cancer. Sedentary lifestyles devoid of regular physical activity predispose individuals to metabolic dysregulation, chronic inflammation, and insulin resistance, creating an environment conducive to tumorigenesis. Moreover, obesity, fueled by the consumption of calorie-dense, nutrient-poor foods, perpetuates a state of chronic low-grade inflammation, fostering the growth and progression of colorectal tumors.

Microbial Mediators: Exploring the Gut Microbiome

Emerging evidence implicates the gut microbiome, a diverse ecosystem of microorganisms residing within the gastrointestinal tract, in colorectal cancer development. Dysbiosis, characterized by an imbalance in microbial composition and function, disrupts the delicate equilibrium between commensal and pathogenic bacteria, triggering inflammatory cascades and promoting carcinogenesis. Furthermore, specific bacterial species, such as Fusobacterium nucleatum and Escherichia coli, have been implicated in the pathogenesis of colorectal cancer, underscoring the intricate relationship between microbial mediators and disease progression.

Inflammatory Instigators: Chronic Inflammation and Colorectal Carcinogenesis

Chronic inflammation, a hallmark of colorectal cancer, fuels the malignant transformation of colonic epithelial cells through the release of pro-inflammatory cytokines and growth factors. Inflammatory bowel diseases (IBD), including ulcerative colitis and Crohn's disease, predispose individuals to an elevated risk of developing colorectal cancer, underscoring the pivotal role of inflammation in disease pathogenesis. Moreover, lifestyle factors such as obesity, smoking, and dietary imbalances perpetuate a state of chronic low-grade inflammation, exacerbating colorectal cancer risk and progression.

Conclusion: Navigating the Complexities of Colorectal Cancer Etiology

In conclusion, colorectal cancer represents a multifaceted disease entity shaped by a complex interplay of genetic, environmental, and lifestyle factors. Understanding the intricate mechanisms underlying its origins is paramount to devising effective preventive strategies and therapeutic interventions to combat this formidable foe. By unraveling the enigma of colorectal cancer etiology, we pave the way for precision medicine approaches tailored to individual risk profiles, ultimately ushering in a new era of personalized oncology. As we continue our quest for knowledge and innovation, let us remain steadfast in our commitment to unraveling the mysteries of colorectal cancer, empowering individuals with the tools needed to navigate the complexities of this disease with resilience and hope.

RISK FACTOR FOR DEVELOPING COLORECTAL CANCER

At the core of colorectal cancer lies a complex interplay of genetic predispositions that confer susceptibility to the disease. Familial adenomatous polyposis (FAP) and Lynch syndrome, two hereditary conditions characterized by mutations in specific genes, significantly elevate the risk of colorectal cancer. Individuals with a family history of these syndromes face a substantially heightened risk and require vigilant monitoring and proactive measures to mitigate potential risks.

Moreover, emerging research has unveiled a myriad of genetic variants associated with increased colorectal cancer susceptibility in the general population. From single nucleotide polymorphisms (SNPs) to chromosomal aberrations, these genetic variations underscore the intricate genetic tapestry that contributes to colorectal cancer risk. Understanding these genetic nuances enables tailored screening and prevention strategies, heralding a paradigm shift towards precision medicine in colorectal cancer management.

Environmental Factors: Navigating the Extrinsic Influences

Beyond genetics, environmental factors wield considerable influence in shaping colorectal cancer risk. Dietary habits, notably those characterized by high consumption of processed meats, red meats, and saturated fats, have emerged as prominent culprits in fueling colorectal carcinogenesis. Conversely, diets rich in fiber, fruits, and vegetables exert protective effects, mitigating the risk of colorectal cancer development.

Environmental exposures, ranging from tobacco smoke to industrial pollutants, also contribute to colorectal cancer risk through mechanisms involving inflammation, oxidative stress, and DNA damage. Furthermore, sedentary lifestyles marked by physical inactivity and prolonged sitting pose additional risk factors, underscoring the pivotal role of lifestyle modifications in colorectal cancer prevention.

Lifestyle Factors: Nurturing Healthful Habits

Lifestyle choices wield profound influence in sculpting colorectal cancer risk trajectories, offering a realm of modifiable factors ripe for intervention. Obesity, a burgeoning epidemic characterized by excessive adiposity, stands as a potent risk factor for colorectal cancer, fostering a pro-inflammatory milieu conducive to tumorigenesis. By adopting healthy eating habits, engaging in regular physical activity, and maintaining a healthy weight, individuals can proactively mitigate colorectal cancer risk and foster overall well-being.

Moreover, the detrimental effects of excessive alcohol consumption on colorectal cancer risk underscore the imperative of moderation in alcohol intake. Alcohol's ability to disrupt cellular homeostasis, promote inflammation, and induce oxidative stress underscores its role as a potent carcinogen in colorectal carcinogenesis. By embracing moderation and practicing responsible alcohol consumption, individuals can attenuate colorectal cancer and safeguard their health.

Conclusion: Empowering Prevention through Knowledge

As we unravel the intricate web of risk factors underpinning colorectal cancer development, a compelling narrative emerges—one of empowerment through knowledge and proactive intervention. Armed with a nuanced understanding of genetic predispositions, environmental influences, and lifestyle choices, individuals possess the tools necessary to chart a course towards colorectal cancer prevention and risk reduction.

By fostering awareness, advocating for lifestyle modifications, and embracing evidence-based screening protocols, we pave the way for a future where colorectal cancer prevalence dwindles, and lives are preserved. Let us embark on this journey together, united in our quest to transcend colorectal cancer's formidable grasp and forge a path towards a future defined by health, resilience, and hope.

SIGNS AND SYMPTOMS

RECOGNISING WARNING SIGNS

Colorectal cancer is often referred to as a "silent killer" due to its potential to develop silently and without noticeable symptoms in the early stages. However, it is crucial to understand that this disease does exhibit warning signs, albeit sometimes subtle or easily overlooked. Recognizing these signs early can significantly improve outcomes by facilitating early diagnosis and intervention.

Common Signs and Symptoms

1. **Changes in Bowel Habits**: One of the most common early signs of colorectal cancer is a change in bowel habits. This may manifest as persistent diarrhea, constipation, or a change in stool consistency that lasts for more than a few days without apparent cause.
2. **Rectal Bleeding or Blood in the Stool**: Any unexplained bleeding from the rectum or blood present in

the stool should be taken seriously. While it may be due to benign conditions such as hemorrhoids, it can also indicate colorectal cancer, especially if it persists or is accompanied by other symptoms.

3. **Abdominal Discomfort or Pain**: Persistent abdominal discomfort, cramping, or pain that does not resolve with over-the-counter remedies warrants investigation. This discomfort may be localized or diffuse and may worsen over time.

4. **Unexplained Weight Loss**: Significant, unintentional weight loss without changes in diet or exercise habits should raise concern, as it can be a sign of various underlying health issues, including colorectal cancer.

5. **Fatigue and Weakness**: Chronic fatigue or weakness that persists despite adequate rest and nutrition may indicate an underlying health problem, including colorectal cancer.

6. **Iron Deficiency Anemia**: Anemia caused by a deficiency in iron may occur in individuals with colorectal cancer due to chronic bleeding from the gastrointestinal tract. Symptoms

may include tiredness, pale skin, and shortness of breath.

7. **Changes in Bowel Urgency or Incomplete Emptying**: A persistent sense of urgency to have a bowel movement or feeling of incomplete emptying after a bowel movement may be indicative of colorectal cancer.

Understanding Red Flags

While some symptoms may seem benign or easily attributable to other causes, certain "red flags" warrant immediate medical attention. These include:

- Unexpected and unexplained changes in bowel habits
- Rectal bleeding or blood in the stool
- Persistent abdominal pain or discomfort
- Unexplained weight loss
- Tiredness that does not improve with rest
- Anemia or symptoms suggestive of significant blood loss
- Any combination of symptoms that persists for more than a few weeks

Conclusion

In conclusion, recognizing the warning signs of colorectal cancer is paramount in the journey towards early detection and effective treatment. By familiarizing ourselves with these signs and symptoms, we empower ourselves and our communities to prioritize proactive health monitoring and seek timely medical evaluation when necessary. Remember, early detection saves lives. Stay vigilant, stay informed, and together, we can overcome the challenges posed by colorectal cancer.

COMMON SYMPTOMS OF COLORECTAL CANCER

Colorectal cancer manifests through a diverse array of symptoms, each harboring its own significance and potential implications. While some symptoms may seem innocuous at first glance, others may herald the presence of a more sinister underlying condition. Therefore, it is paramount to approach the assessment of symptoms with a discerning eye, recognizing the subtle nuances that may betray the presence of colorectal cancer.

Unraveling the Spectrum of Symptoms

1. Changes in Bowel Habits

One of the earliest and most commonly reported symptoms of colorectal cancer is a change in bowel habits. Individuals may notice alterations in the frequency, consistency, or caliber of their bowel movements. These changes may manifest as persistent diarrhea, constipation, or alternating episodes of both. Moreover, individuals may experience a sense of incomplete evacuation or a feeling of urgency despite minimal stool passage.

2. Rectal Bleeding

Rectal bleeding, often characterized by the presence of blood in the stool or on toilet paper, is another hallmark symptom of colorectal cancer. While hemorrhoids and anal fissures may account for benign causes of rectal bleeding, the persistence or worsening of this symptom warrants further investigation to rule out underlying malignancies.

3. Abdominal Discomfort and Pain

The presence of persistent abdominal discomfort, cramping, or pain may signify the presence of colorectal cancer, particularly as the tumor grows and exerts pressure on surrounding tissues and organs. Individuals may describe a dull ache or a sense of fullness in the abdomen, which may be accompanied by bloating or a feeling of abdominal distension.

4. Unexplained Weight Loss

Unintentional weight loss, often defined as a loss of more than 5% of body weight within a span of six months to a year, can be a concerning indicator of underlying malignancy, including colorectal cancer. This weight loss may occur despite a stable or increased appetite, and it is often accompanied by fatigue, weakness, and a general decline in overall health.

5. Fatigue and Weakness

The onset of unexplained fatigue and weakness, which persist despite an adequate amount of rest and sleep, may signify the presence of colorectal cancer. This fatigue may be attributed to anemia resulting from chronic blood loss, nutritional deficiencies, or the metabolic demands imposed by the growing tumor.

6. Changes in Bowel Movement Sensation

Individuals may experience changes in the sensation of bowel movements, such as a feeling of incomplete evacuation, tenesmus (a persistent urge to defecate), or the sensation of obstruction or blockage within the rectum or colon. These sensations may be indicative of the presence of a tumor or mass obstructing the bowel lumen.

7. Iron Deficiency Anemia

Iron deficiency anemia, characterized by a decrease in the body's red blood cell count and hemoglobin levels due to insufficient iron stores, may occur as a consequence of chronic blood loss associated with colorectal cancer. Individuals may present with symptoms such as pallor, weakness, shortness of breath, and palpitations, prompting further investigation into the underlying cause.

Recognizing the Importance of Early Detection

The timely recognition and evaluation of colorectal cancer symptoms play a pivotal role in facilitating early detection and intervention, thereby improving treatment outcomes and prognosis. As such, individuals are encouraged to remain vigilant and proactive in monitoring their health and promptly report any concerning symptoms to their healthcare providers. Moreover, healthcare professionals are urged to maintain a high index of suspicion for colorectal cancer, particularly in individuals with risk factors predisposing them to the development of this disease.

Conclusion: Empowering Individuals Through Knowledge

In conclusion, the spectrum of symptoms associated with colorectal cancer serves as a silent yet powerful indicator of the presence of this disease. By familiarizing themselves with these symptoms and remaining vigilant in their recognition, individuals can take proactive steps towards early detection and intervention, ultimately enhancing their chances of successful treatment and recovery. Through the dissemination of knowledge and awareness, we empower individuals to confront colorectal cancer with resilience, determination, and hope.

As we navigate the complexities of colorectal cancer symptoms, let us heed the call to vigilance, for within the subtleties of these silent indicators lies the potential to unravel the mysteries of this formidable adversary and emerge victorious in the fight against cancer.

WHEN TO SEEK MEDICAL ATTENTION

Colorectal cancer, notorious for its silent progression, gradually reveals itself through a myriad of signs and symptoms, each holding invaluable insights into the state of one's health. From changes in bowel habits and rectal bleeding to persistent abdominal discomfort and unexplained weight loss, these subtle clues serve as frontline indicators of potential malignancy lurking within the colon or rectum. However, recognizing these signs requires a keen eye and a willingness to confront the possibility of colorectal cancer, prompting individuals to take proactive measures to seek timely medical attention.

The Importance of Early Detection:

Early detection remains the cornerstone in the battle against colorectal cancer, offering individuals the best chance for successful treatment and improved outcomes. By recognizing the signs and symptoms early on and promptly seeking medical evaluation, individuals can undergo timely screenings, diagnostic tests, and interventions that may ultimately save lives. Hence, the significance of understanding when to seek medical attention cannot be overstated, as it serves as a pivotal step towards early detection and potentially life-saving interventions.

Navigating the Gray Areas:

Despite the clarity of certain signs and symptoms, navigating the gray areas of colorectal cancer detection can prove challenging for many individuals. Symptoms such as abdominal discomfort, fatigue, and changes in appetite may often be dismissed as common ailments or attributed to other benign causes, leading to delays in seeking medical evaluation. Thus, it becomes imperative to educate individuals on the subtle nuances of colorectal cancer symptoms, encouraging them to remain vigilant and proactive in addressing any concerning changes in their health.

Empowering Individuals to Take Action:

In the quest for early detection and intervention, empowering individuals to take action becomes paramount. Through education, awareness campaigns, and proactive healthcare initiatives, individuals can be equipped with the knowledge and resources needed to recognize potential signs and symptoms of colorectal cancer and take prompt action to seek medical attention. By fostering a culture of health literacy and empowerment, we can cultivate a society where early detection becomes the norm rather than the exception, ultimately saving lives and reducing the burden of colorectal cancer on individuals and communities alike.

Conclusion:

In conclusion, the signs and symptoms of colorectal cancer serve as invaluable indicators of potential malignancy within the colon or rectum. By understanding the significance of these subtle clues and knowing when to seek medical attention, individuals can take proactive steps towards early detection and intervention, ultimately improving their chances for successful treatment and survival. Therefore, let us heed the call to action, empower ourselves and others with knowledge, and strive towards a future where colorectal cancer is detected early, treated effectively, and overcome with resilience and hope.

DIAGNOSIS

SCREENING GUIDELINES AND RECOMMENDATIONS

Before delving into diagnosis, it's crucial to grasp the essence of colorectal cancer. Originating in the colon or rectum, this malignancy arises from the uncontrolled growth of abnormal cells. Risk factors encompass lifestyle choices, genetic predisposition, and age, underscoring the multifaceted nature of its etiology. Colorectal cancer often manifests insidiously, emphasizing the significance of proactive screening initiatives to intercept its progression at early stages.

Screening Guidelines and Recommendations:

1. **Population-Based Screening Initiatives:**
   - National and international health organizations advocate for population-based screening programs to mitigate colorectal cancer. These initiatives aim to

target asymptomatic individuals at average risk, fostering early detection and intervention.

- o Recommended screening modalities vary across jurisdictions, with colonoscopy, fecal occult blood testing (FOBT), fecal immunochemical testing (FIT), and sigmoidoscopy constituting the primary options. Guidelines emphasize the importance of selecting an appropriate screening modality based on individual risk profiles, preferences, and resource availability.

2. **Age-Based Screening Recommendations:**

- o Age represents a significant determinant in colorectal cancer screening recommendations. Most guidelines advocate initiating screening at age 50 for average-risk individuals, although earlier initiation may be warranted for high-risk cohorts.

- o The American Cancer Society, U.S. Preventive Services Task Force, and European Society of Gastrointestinal Endoscopy delineate age-specific screening protocols, tailoring recommendations to optimize efficacy and resource allocation.

3. **High-Risk Population Screening:**
   - o High-risk populations, including individuals with a family history of colorectal cancer, hereditary syndromes (e.g., Lynch syndrome), or predisposing conditions (e.g., inflammatory bowel disease), necessitate tailored screening strategies.
   - o Genetic counseling and testing play a pivotal role in identifying high-risk individuals, facilitating personalized screening regimens and preventive interventions.

4. **Screening Modalities:**
   - o Colonoscopy, the gold standard for colorectal cancer screening,

- enables direct visualization of the colon and rectum, facilitating polyp detection and biopsy procurement.
  - Stool-based tests, encompassing FOBT and FIT, offer non-invasive alternatives for colorectal cancer screening, detecting occult blood indicative of underlying pathology.
  - Emerging modalities, including virtual colonoscopy (CT colonography) and stool DNA testing, exhibit promise in enhancing screening accessibility and compliance, albeit warranting further validation and standardization.

Conclusion:

In conclusion, effective colorectal cancer diagnosis hinges on adherence to established screening guidelines and recommendations. By embracing a multifaceted approach encompassing population-based initiatives, age-specific protocols, and tailored strategies for high-risk cohorts, healthcare stakeholders can foster early detection and mitigate disease burden. It is imperative to prioritize awareness, education, and accessibility to screening modalities, thereby empowering individuals to embark on a proactive journey towards colorectal cancer prevention and early intervention. Together, let us illuminate the path towards a future where colorectal cancer is detected early, treated effectively, and ultimately, conquered.

TYPES OF SCREENING TEST

Colorectal cancer is the third most common cancer diagnosed in both men and women worldwide, with significant morbidity and mortality rates. However, when detected early, the five-year survival rate can exceed 90%. This highlights the critical importance of screening in the fight against colorectal cancer. Screening tests are designed to detect abnormalities in the colon or rectum before symptoms manifest, allowing for early intervention and improved outcomes.

Types of Screening Tests:

1. **Fecal Occult Blood Test (FOBT):**
   - This non-invasive test detects the presence of blood in the stool, which may indicate the presence of colorectal polyps or cancer.
   - FOBT can be performed at home using a stool sample kit, making it convenient and accessible for many individuals.
   - However, it is important to note that FOBT may yield false-positive results, leading to unnecessary anxiety and further testing.
2. **Fecal Immunochemical Test (FIT):**
   - Similar to FOBT, FIT detects blood in the stool, but it is more specific for human hemoglobin, reducing the likelihood of false-positive results.
   - FIT is also performed using a stool sample kit and offers a simple and cost-effective screening option.

- o Due to its higher specificity, FIT may be preferred over FOBT in some settings.

3. **Colonoscopy:**
   - o Colonoscopy is considered the gold standard for colorectal cancer screening, offering both diagnostic and therapeutic capabilities.
   - o During a colonoscopy, a flexible tube with a camera is inserted into the colon, allowing for visualization of the entire colon and rectum.
   - o In addition to detecting cancer, colonoscopy can also identify and remove precancerous polyps, potentially preventing the development of cancer altogether.
   - o While colonoscopy is highly effective, it requires bowel preparation and sedation, and some individuals may experience discomfort or complications.

4. **Flexible Sigmoidoscopy:**
   - o Similar to colonoscopy, flexible sigmoidoscopy involves

inserting a flexible tube into the rectum and lower colon to examine for abnormalities.

- o However, flexible sigmoidoscopy only examines the lower part of the colon, whereas colonoscopy examines the entire colon.
- o This procedure may be less invasive than colonoscopy, but it has limitations in its ability to detect abnormalities in the upper colon.

5. **Virtual Colonoscopy (CT Colonography):**
   - o Virtual colonoscopy utilizes computed tomography (CT) imaging to create detailed images of the colon and rectum.
   - o It offers a less invasive alternative to traditional colonoscopy, as it does not require the insertion of a scope into the colon.
   - o However, virtual colonoscopy still requires bowel preparation and may involve exposure to radiation.

Choosing the Right Test:

The choice of screening test depends on various factors, including individual preferences, risk factors, and medical history. Factors such as age, family history of colorectal cancer, and the presence of symptoms may also influence the selection of the most appropriate screening test. It is essential to discuss screening options with a healthcare provider to determine the best course of action based on individual circumstances.

Conclusion:

Colorectal cancer screening tests play a critical role in early detection and prevention, offering individuals the opportunity for timely intervention and improved outcomes. By understanding the different types of screening tests available, individuals can make informed decisions about their health and well-being. It is imperative to prioritize regular screening and engage in open communication with healthcare providers to ensure optimal colorectal cancer prevention and management strategies. Together, let us continue to advance in the fight against colorectal cancer through education, awareness, and early detection.

DIAGNOSTIC PROCEDURES FOR CONFIRMING DIAGNOSIS

The journey towards defeating colorectal cancer begins with an accurate diagnosis. With advancements in medical science, diagnostic procedures have evolved, offering clinicians an array of tools to confirm the presence of colorectal cancer with precision. In this note, we embark on a journey through the diagnostic landscape, uncovering the methodologies that underpin the process of confirming colorectal cancer diagnosis.

Colonoscopy: Peering into the Depths

Colonoscopy stands as a cornerstone in the diagnosis of colorectal cancer. This procedure involves the insertion of a flexible, slender tube equipped with a camera into the rectum and colon. Through real-time visualization, clinicians can examine the lining of the colon for abnormalities such as polyps or tumors.

Additionally, tissue samples, known as biopsies, may be obtained during colonoscopy for further analysis. With its ability to provide direct visualization and biopsy procurement, colonoscopy remains the gold standard for diagnosing colorectal cancer.

Virtual Colonoscopy: Unveiling a Digital Frontier

Innovations in medical imaging have birthed the concept of virtual colonoscopy, also known as CT colonography. This non-invasive procedure utilizes computed tomography (CT) scans to generate detailed, three-dimensional images of the colon and rectum. Unlike traditional colonoscopy, virtual colonoscopy does not require sedation or the insertion of a colonoscope. Instead, patients undergo a CT scan, and the images are processed to create a virtual representation of the colon. Virtual colonoscopy offers a less invasive alternative for individuals who may be hesitant to undergo traditional colonoscopy while still providing accurate visualization of the colon and detection of abnormalities.

Fecal Occult Blood Test (FOBT): Detecting Hidden Traces

The fecal occult blood test (FOBT) serves as a screening tool for detecting occult (hidden) blood in the stool, which may indicate the presence of colorectal cancer or precancerous polyps. During the test, patients collect stool samples at home and submit them to a laboratory for analysis. FOBT can help identify individuals who may require further diagnostic evaluation, such as a colonoscopy, for a definitive diagnosis. While FOBT is less invasive than other diagnostic procedures, its sensitivity and specificity may vary, and false-positive results can occur, necessitating confirmatory testing.

Flexible Sigmoidoscopy: A Focused Examination

Flexible sigmoidoscopy involves the insertion of a flexible, lighted tube into the rectum and lower portion of the colon (sigmoid colon) to visualize and examine the colonic mucosa for abnormalities. While similar to colonoscopy, flexible sigmoidoscopy provides a more limited view of the colon and is primarily used to evaluate the lower portion of the colon. This procedure may be recommended as a screening tool for individuals at average risk of colorectal cancer or as a diagnostic tool for individuals with symptoms localized to the lower colon.

Genetic Testing: Deciphering the Code

Advancements in molecular biology have paved the way for genetic testing in the diagnosis of colorectal cancer. Genetic testing involves analyzing a patient's DNA to identify specific genetic mutations or alterations associated with an increased risk of developing colorectal cancer. Individuals with a family history of colorectal cancer or certain hereditary cancer syndromes may undergo genetic testing to assess their risk and inform personalized screening and management strategies. Additionally, genetic testing may be used to guide treatment decisions, particularly in the era of precision medicine, where targeted therapies are tailored to the genetic profile of the tumor.

Conclusion:

As we conclude our exploration of diagnostic procedures for a confirming colorectal cancer diagnosis, we are reminded of the critical role that precision plays in the fight against this formidable disease. From traditional colonoscopy to cutting-edge genetic testing, each diagnostic tool serves as a beacon of hope, guiding clinicians towards early detection and intervention. As we continue to advance on the frontier of medical innovation, may we harness the power of these diagnostic methodologies to illuminate the path towards improved outcomes and, ultimately, the eradication of colorectal cancer.

STAGES OF COLORECTAL CANCER

EXPLANING THE TNM STAGING SYSTEM

The TNM staging system provides a standardized method for describing the extent of primary tumor (T), regional lymph node involvement (N), and distant metastasis (M). This alphanumeric classification system offers a systematic approach to assessing the progression and spread of colorectal cancer, facilitating accurate communication among healthcare professionals, and guiding treatment strategies.

T Stage: Assessing the Primary Tumor:

The T stage reflects the size and extent of the primary tumor within the colon or rectum. It categorizes tumors based on their invasion depth into the layers of the intestinal wall. Tumor size, depth of invasion, and involvement of adjacent structures dictate T stage classification. T stages range from Tis (carcinoma in situ) to T4b (tumor penetrates the visceral peritoneum or directly invades adjacent organs or structures).

N Stage: Evaluating Regional Lymph Node Involvement:

Regional lymph node involvement serves as a crucial prognostic factor in colorectal cancer. The N stage characterizes the presence and extent of tumor spread to nearby lymph nodes. Assessment of lymph node involvement involves careful examination of surgically resected specimens and imaging studies. N stages range from N0 (no regional lymph node metastasis) to N2 (metastasis in four or more regional lymph nodes).

M Stage: Detecting Distant Metastasis:

Distant metastasis signifies the spread of colorectal cancer beyond the confines of the colon and regional lymph nodes to distant organs or tissues. The M stage encompasses a comprehensive evaluation of distant metastatic sites, including the liver, lungs, bones, and other distant organs. Accurate detection of distant metastasis is vital for determining treatment options and predicting overall survival.

Clinical Implications of TNM Staging in Colorectal Cancer:

The TNM staging system serves as a pivotal tool in clinical decision-making for colorectal cancer management. It guides treatment selection, surgical planning, and the determination of adjuvant therapies. Additionally, TNM staging facilitates risk stratification, enabling healthcare providers to tailor interventions based on individual patient characteristics and disease severity.

Prognostic Value and Survival Outcomes:

TNM staging provides valuable prognostic information, aiding in the prediction of patient outcomes and survival probabilities. Higher TNM stages correlate with increased tumor burden and a poorer prognosis. Survival rates progressively decline with advancing TNM stages, highlighting the critical importance of early detection and intervention.

Challenges and Limitations:

Despite its utility, the TNM staging system possesses certain limitations and challenges. Variability in tumor sampling, imaging modalities, and interpretation criteria may introduce inconsistencies in staging accuracy. Moreover, the TNM system primarily relies on anatomical factors, potentially overlooking important biological and molecular characteristics influencing tumor behavior.

Future Directions:

Advancements in imaging technology, molecular profiling, and precision medicine hold promise for refining colorectal cancer staging and enhancing prognostic accuracy. Integrating molecular biomarkers and genetic signatures into existing staging systems may improve risk stratification and treatment selection, paving the way for personalized therapeutic approaches.

Conclusion:

The TNM staging system stands as a cornerstone in the management of colorectal cancer, offering a standardized framework for assessing tumor extent and guiding therapeutic decisions. By comprehensively evaluating the primary tumor, regional lymph nodes, and distant metastasis, the TNM staging system provides invaluable prognostic information essential for optimizing patient care. As we continue to unravel the complexities of colorectal cancer, the TNM staging system remains a vital tool in our quest to combat this formidable disease, guiding us toward improved outcomes and enhanced survival for patients worldwide.

UNDERSTANDING THE FOUR STAGES OF COLORECTAL CANCER

Stage 0: Understanding the Precursor

At the outset of our journey lies Stage 0, often referred to as carcinoma in situ. This stage represents the earliest form of colorectal cancer, where abnormal cells are confined to the inner lining of the colon or rectum. Despite its localized nature, Stage 0 serves as a crucial indicator of potential progression to invasive cancer if left untreated. Understanding the significance of early detection and intervention is paramount at this stage, as it offers the opportunity for curative treatments such as endoscopic resection or surgical excision. By recognizing Stage 0 as the precursor to more advanced forms of colorectal cancer, we underscore the importance of proactive screening and surveillance efforts in preventing disease progression and preserving long-term health.

Stage I: Embracing Localized Growth

As we progress along the continuum of colorectal cancer staging, we encounter Stage I, characterized by the localized growth of cancerous cells within the colon or rectum. At this stage, the tumor has penetrated beyond the inner lining but remains confined to the mucosa or submucosa, with no involvement of nearby lymph nodes or distant organs. Despite its relatively contained nature, Stage I colorectal cancer poses significant challenges and considerations for patients and healthcare providers. Surgical resection serves as the primary treatment modality, with the potential for adjuvant therapies such as chemotherapy or radiation depending on individual risk factors and tumor characteristics. By embracing the concept of localized growth in Stage I colorectal cancer, we emphasize the importance of multidisciplinary care and informed decision-making in optimizing patient outcomes and minimizing disease recurrence.

Stage II: Confronting Regional Invasion

Moving forward in our exploration, we confront Stage II colorectal cancer, marked by the invasion of cancer cells into the muscular layers of the colon or rectum. At this critical juncture, the disease extends beyond the confines of the primary tumor yet remains localized within the bowel wall without lymph node involvement or distant metastasis. The management of Stage II colorectal cancer presents a complex interplay of clinical, pathological, and prognostic factors, necessitating a tailored approach to treatment and surveillance. Surgical resection remains the cornerstone of therapy, often supplemented by adjuvant chemotherapy or radiation in select cases.

However, the decision to pursue additional treatments must be weighed carefully against the potential risks and benefits, considering factors such as tumor grade, lymphovascular invasion, and patient comorbidities. By confronting the challenges of regional invasion in Stage II colorectal cancer, we underscore the importance of individualized care and shared decision-making in optimizing patient outcomes and quality of life.

Stage III: Grappling with Lymphatic Involvement

As we reach the pinnacle of our journey, we confront Stage III colorectal cancer, characterized by the involvement of nearby lymph nodes in the spread of cancerous cells. At this advanced stage, the disease transcends the confines of the primary tumor and infiltrates the lymphatic system, posing significant challenges and complexities in its management. Surgical resection remains a cornerstone of therapy, often supplemented by adjuvant chemotherapy or radiation to target residual cancer cells and reduce the risk of recurrence. However, the presence of lymphatic involvement introduces additional considerations for treatment planning and prognostication, necessitating a multidisciplinary approach and ongoing surveillance. By grappling with the complexities of lymphatic involvement in Stage III colorectal cancer, we underscore the importance of comprehensive care and vigilant monitoring in achieving optimal outcomes and long-term survivorship.

Conclusion:

In conclusion, the staging of colorectal cancer serves as a cornerstone of patient care, guiding treatment decisions, prognostication, and surveillance strategies. Through our exploration of the four stages of colorectal cancer, we have gained invaluable insight into the progression of this disease and the challenges it presents for patients and healthcare providers alike. By understanding the significance of each stage and its implications for management, we empower individuals to navigate the complexities of colorectal cancer with knowledge, resilience, and hope. As we continue to advance in our understanding and treatment of this disease, let us remain steadfast in our commitment to improving outcomes and enhancing the lives of those affected by colorectal cancer.

PROGNOSIS AND SURVIVAL RATE

To comprehend the prognosis and survival rates associated with colorectal cancer, one must first grasp the concept of cancer staging. The staging system provides a standardized framework for categorizing the extent of cancer spread, facilitating communication among healthcare providers, and guiding treatment decisions. In colorectal cancer, staging typically follows the TNM system, which evaluates the primary tumor (T), regional lymph nodes (N), and distant metastasis (M).

Stage 0: At this earliest stage, cancerous cells are confined to the innermost layer of the colon or rectum's lining, known as the mucosa. Also referred to as carcinoma in situ, stage 0 colorectal cancer holds a favorable prognosis with high survival rates following surgical resection.

Stage I: Cancer has penetrated beyond the mucosa into the submucosa, or muscle layer, of the colon or rectum wall. Despite the presence of cancerous cells in nearby tissues, stage I colorectal cancer is considered localized and often curable with surgery alone.

Stage II: In this stage, cancer has invaded through the muscle layer into the outermost layers of the colon or rectum but has not yet spread to nearby lymph nodes or distant organs. While the prognosis for stage II colorectal cancer varies depending on factors such as tumor size and grade, surgical intervention remains the primary treatment modality.

Stage III: Characterized by the presence of cancer cells in nearby lymph nodes, stage III colorectal cancer represents regional spread beyond the primary tumor site. Treatment typically involves a combination of surgery, chemotherapy, and possibly radiation therapy, with the aim of eradicating cancer cells and reducing the risk of recurrence.

Stage IV: At this advanced stage, cancer has metastasized to distant organs or tissues, such as the liver, lungs, or peritoneum. While stage IV colorectal cancer poses significant challenges, advancements in systemic therapies, including targeted therapies and immunotherapy, have improved survival outcomes for some patients.

Prognosis and Survival Rates

The prognosis for colorectal cancer is influenced by various factors, including the cancer stage, tumor characteristics, patient demographics, and treatment response. Survival rates are often expressed as five-year relative survival rates, which estimate the percentage of patients who are alive five years after diagnosis compared to the general population.

Stage 0 and I: With cancer confined to the inner layers of the colon or rectum, the five-year relative survival rates for stage 0 and stage I colorectal cancer exceed 90%, highlighting the favorable outcomes associated with early-stage disease detection and intervention.

Stage II: Despite the absence of lymph node involvement, stage II colorectal cancer carries a variable prognosis, with five-year relative survival rates ranging from 60% to 80%. Factors such as tumor size, location, and histology may influence individual prognosis and treatment decisions.

Stage III: The presence of cancer cells in nearby lymph nodes significantly impacts prognosis, with five-year relative survival rates ranging from approximately 40% to 70% for stage III colorectal cancer. Adjuvant chemotherapy following surgical resection plays a crucial role in reducing the risk of disease recurrence and improving long-term outcomes.

Stage IV: Advanced-stage colorectal cancer presents formidable challenges, with five-year relative survival rates typically ranging from 10% to 20%. However, individual prognosis can vary widely based on factors such as the extent of metastatic spread, tumor biology, treatment response, and overall health status.

Conclusion

As we conclude our exploration of the stages of colorectal cancer and their implications for prognosis and survival, it is evident that early detection, accurate staging, and personalized treatment are essential in optimizing patient outcomes. While the journey through colorectal cancer may be fraught with challenges, advancements in screening, diagnostics, and therapeutics offer hope for improved survival and quality of life. By fostering a collaborative approach among patients, caregivers, and healthcare providers, we can navigate the complexities of colorectal cancer with resilience, compassion, and unwavering determination.

TREATMENT OPTIONS

SURGERY: RESECTION AND ANASTOMOSIS

In the realm of combating colorectal cancer, surgery stands as a stalwart guardian, wielding the power to excise the malignant invader and restore hope to those afflicted. Among the myriad treatment options available, surgical intervention, particularly resection and anastomosis, emerges as a cornerstone of curative efforts. In this comprehensive exploration, we embark on a journey through the intricate world of colorectal cancer surgery, unraveling its complexities, nuances, and transformative potential.

Understanding Colorectal Cancer Surgery:

At the heart of colorectal cancer surgery lies the principle of excising the tumor along with a margin of healthy tissue to ensure complete eradication. Resection, the primary surgical approach, involves removing the affected portion of the colon or rectum, aiming to eliminate all traces of cancerous growth. Following resection, anastomosis, the process of reconnecting the remaining healthy segments of the intestine, facilitates the restoration of intestinal continuity and function.

The Surgical Landscape:

Within the realm of colorectal cancer surgery, various approaches and techniques abound, each tailored to the unique characteristics of the disease and the individual patient. From traditional open surgery to minimally invasive laparoscopic and robotic-assisted procedures, the surgical landscape offers a spectrum of options, each with its own merits and considerations.

Precision and Expertise:

Central to the success of colorectal cancer surgery are the skillful hands and discerning eyes of the surgical team. Surgeons, armed with years of specialized training and experience, navigate the intricacies of anatomy with precision and finesse, ensuring optimal outcomes for their patients. Collaborating seamlessly with an interdisciplinary team of healthcare professionals, including oncologists, radiologists, and nurses, they orchestrate a symphony of care aimed at delivering excellence at every turn.

Navigating the Treatment Journey:

For patients facing colorectal cancer surgery, the journey is marked by a blend of apprehension, hope, and resilience. From the initial consultation and diagnostic workup to the meticulous planning and execution of the surgical procedure, every step of the treatment journey is imbued with a sense of purpose and determination. Supported by a network of caregivers, loved ones, and healthcare providers, patients traverse the path towards healing with courage and fortitude.

Beyond the Operating Room:

While surgery serves as a potent weapon against colorectal cancer, its impact extends far beyond the confines of the operating room. For many patients, the road to recovery encompasses a multifaceted approach, incorporating postoperative care, rehabilitation, and ongoing surveillance. With steadfast commitment and unwavering dedication, patients and healthcare professionals alike collaborate to ensure optimal outcomes and long-term success.

Embracing Innovation and Advancement:

In the ever-evolving landscape of colorectal cancer treatment, innovation and advancement pave the way forward, heralding new possibilities and opportunities for progress. From groundbreaking surgical techniques to cutting-edge technologies and therapies, the future holds promise for continued refinement and enhancement of surgical outcomes. Embracing a spirit of innovation and collaboration, the medical community remains steadfast in its pursuit of excellence and innovation in the fight against colorectal cancer.

A Message of Hope:

As we navigate the complexities of colorectal cancer surgery, let us not forget the essence of hope that underpins every endeavor. In the face of adversity, hope serves as a beacon of light, guiding us through the darkest of times and inspiring us to persevere against all odds. With each surgical incision and every suture placed, let us reaffirm our commitment to healing, resilience, and the unwavering pursuit of a brighter tomorrow.

Conclusion:

In closing, the journey through colorectal cancer surgery is one fraught with challenges, triumphs, and moments of profound significance. From the operating room to the halls of recovery, each step along the way serves as a testament to the indomitable spirit of the human experience. As we forge ahead, let us embrace the transformative power of surgery, harnessing its potential to heal, restore, and renew. Together, let us chart a course towards a future free from the scourge of colorectal cancer, guided by a shared commitment to excellence, compassion, and hope.

CHEMOTHERAPHY: HOW IT WORKS AND SIDE EFFECTS

Chemotherapy stands as one of the formidable weapons in the arsenal against colorectal cancer, offering hope and promise in the battle against this relentless disease. In this comprehensive exploration, we delve into the intricate mechanisms, profound efficacy, and nuanced side effects of chemotherapy, shedding light on its pivotal role in the fight for survival.

At its core, chemotherapy operates on the principle of targeting rapidly dividing cells, a hallmark characteristic of cancer cells. By disrupting the cell cycle and inhibiting proliferation, chemotherapy agents aim to thwart the relentless growth of cancerous tissues, thereby impeding tumor progression and metastasis. Through a meticulous understanding of cellular biology and pharmacokinetics, researchers have meticulously crafted a diverse array of chemotherapy drugs, each with its own unique mechanism of action and therapeutic profile.

COLORECTAL CANCER

One of the cornerstones of chemotherapy in colorectal cancer treatment is the utilization of cytotoxic agents such as fluorouracil (5-FU), oxaliplatin, and irinotecan. These drugs exert their anti-cancer effects through various mechanisms, including interference with DNA synthesis, induction of DNA damage, and disruption of microtubule function. Combinations of these agents, administered in carefully orchestrated regimens, have demonstrated remarkable efficacy in both adjuvant and palliative settings, offering patients a lifeline amidst the turmoil of cancer diagnosis.

However, alongside its formidable efficacy, chemotherapy also unfurls a tapestry of side effects that can challenge patients physically, emotionally, and psychologically. From the ubiquitous nausea and vomiting to the debilitating fatigue and myelosuppression, the toll exacted by chemotherapy is profound and multifaceted. Neuropathy, mucositis, alopecia, and cognitive impairment stand as poignant reminders of the sacrifices endured in the pursuit of survival.

Yet, amidst the adversity, there exists a beacon of hope—a testament to the resilience of the human spirit and the strides made in supportive care. Antiemetics, growth factors, and neuropathic agents serve as indispensable allies, ameliorating the burdensome side effects and enhancing patients' quality of life. Moreover, advancements in personalized medicine and targeted therapies herald a new era of precision oncology, promising to mitigate toxicity while maximizing therapeutic efficacy.

As we navigate the intricate landscape of chemotherapy in colorectal cancer treatment, it is imperative to recognize the profound impact it exerts not only on tumor burden but also on the lives of patients and their loved ones. Each infusion embodies a testament to courage, resilience, and unwavering determination—a poignant reminder of the indomitable human spirit in the face of adversity.

In closing, let us embrace the promise of chemotherapy with tempered optimism and unwavering resolve, recognizing its pivotal role in the fight against colorectal cancer.

Together, through collaboration, innovation, and compassion, we can forge a path towards a future where cancer is not a formidable foe but a conquerable adversary—a future where hope reigns supreme and survival knows no bounds.

RADIATION THERAPHY: BENEFITS AND RISKS

Radiation therapy stands as a beacon of hope in the treatment landscape for colorectal cancer, offering a potent weapon against the insidious progression of this disease. Within the realms of oncology, its utilization represents a pivotal moment in the battle against cancerous cells, wielding both benefits and risks that demand careful consideration. In this comprehensive exploration, we embark on a journey through the intricate terrain of radiation therapy, illuminating its efficacy, challenges, and transformative potential in the context of colorectal cancer treatment.

Understanding Radiation Therapy:

Radiation therapy, also known as radiotherapy, operates on the principle of delivering high-energy radiation beams to targeted areas of the body afflicted by cancer. This targeted approach aims to destroy cancer cells or impede their growth, thereby mitigating tumor progression and offering the prospect of remission or symptom alleviation. In the realm of colorectal cancer, radiation therapy finds application across various stages of the disease, serving as an adjunct to surgical interventions, a primary treatment modality, or a palliative measure to alleviate symptoms and improve quality of life.

Benefits of Radiation Therapy:

The benefits of radiation therapy in the treatment of colorectal cancer are manifold, encompassing both curative and palliative objectives. As a curative modality, radiation therapy plays a vital role in neoadjuvant or adjuvant settings, shrinking tumors prior to surgery to facilitate resection or eradicating residual cancer cells postoperatively to minimize the risk of recurrence. Additionally, in cases where surgical intervention may not be feasible due to tumor location or patient factors, radiation therapy assumes a primary curative role, offering the prospect of tumor control and disease management.

Furthermore, radiation therapy serves as a potent tool in palliative care, ameliorating symptoms such as pain, bleeding, and obstruction in advanced colorectal cancer cases. By targeting cancerous lesions or metastases, radiation therapy can effectively alleviate distressing symptoms, enhance patient comfort, and optimize quality of life, thereby bestowing invaluable relief upon individuals confronting the burdens of advanced disease.

Risks and Challenges:

Despite its profound therapeutic potential, radiation therapy entails inherent risks and challenges that necessitate meticulous evaluation and management. Foremost among these is the risk of radiation-induced toxicity, which may manifest as acute or chronic side effects affecting normal tissues surrounding the targeted area. Gastrointestinal toxicity, encompassing symptoms such as nausea, diarrhea, and rectal irritation, represents a common challenge in the context of colorectal cancer radiation therapy, necessitating vigilant monitoring and supportive care interventions.

Moreover, radiation therapy carries the risk of long-term complications, including bowel dysfunction, urinary disturbances, and sexual dysfunction, which may significantly impact patient quality of life post-treatment. Additionally, there exists a risk of radiation-induced secondary malignancies, albeit rare, necessitating judicious consideration of treatment indications, radiation dose optimization, and follow-up surveillance protocols to mitigate this potential hazard.

Navigating the Path Forward

In navigating the complexities of radiation therapy in the treatment of colorectal cancer, a multidisciplinary approach emerges as paramount, encompassing collaboration among oncologists, radiation oncologists, surgeons, and allied healthcare professionals. Through comprehensive pretreatment assessment, individualized treatment planning, and vigilant toxicity management, the therapeutic efficacy of radiation therapy can be maximized while minimizing the associated risks and optimizing patient outcomes.

Furthermore, ongoing research endeavors continue to advance the field of radiation therapy, unraveling novel techniques such as intensity-modulated radiation therapy (IMRT), stereotactic body radiation therapy (SBRT), and proton beam therapy, which hold promise in enhancing treatment precision, minimizing toxicity, and expanding therapeutic options for colorectal cancer patients.

Conclusion:

In the realm of colorectal cancer treatment, radiation therapy stands as a potent ally, offering a multifaceted approach to combating this formidable adversary. Through its curative and palliative applications, radiation therapy holds the potential to instill hope, alleviate suffering, and transform the trajectory of disease for countless individuals confronting the challenges of colorectal cancer. By embracing a nuanced understanding of its benefits and risks, alongside a commitment to interdisciplinary collaboration and innovation, we illuminate the path forward towards realizing the promise of radiation therapy in the pursuit of healing and restoration.

IMMUNOTHERAPHY AND TARGETED THERAPIES

Immunotherapy, often hailed as the "fifth pillar" of cancer treatment, harnesses the body's immune system to recognize and attack cancer cells. Unlike conventional therapies, which directly target cancer cells, immunotherapy stimulates the immune system to identify and destroy tumors while sparing healthy tissues. From checkpoint inhibitors to adoptive cell therapies, a diverse array of immunotherapeutic strategies is revolutionizing cancer treatment paradigms. We delve into the mechanisms behind these therapies, exploring their successes, challenges, and potential applications in colorectal cancer management.

Unraveling Targeted Therapies:

Targeted therapies represent a precision approach to cancer treatment, aiming to disrupt specific molecules or pathways involved in tumor growth and progression. By honing in on the unique genetic alterations or molecular signatures of cancer cells, targeted therapies offer the promise of personalized and more effective treatment options. From monoclonal antibodies to small molecule inhibitors, we explore the intricacies of targeted therapies, highlighting their mechanisms of action, clinical efficacy, and evolving landscape in colorectal cancer therapeutics.

Navigating the Clinical Landscape:

While immunotherapy and targeted therapies hold immense promise, navigating the clinical landscape requires a nuanced understanding of patient selection, treatment regimens, and potential adverse effects. We delve into the clinical trials and research endeavors shaping the development and refinement of these therapies, shedding light on the criteria for patient eligibility, treatment response assessment, and ongoing efforts to optimize outcomes. Through case studies and real-world examples, we elucidate the practical implications of incorporating immunotherapy and targeted therapies into the multimodal management of colorectal cancer.

Challenges and Opportunities:

Despite the remarkable progress witnessed in the field of immunotherapy and targeted therapies, challenges persist on the road to widespread implementation and efficacy. From innate and acquired resistance mechanisms to immune-related adverse events, we confront the hurdles that hinder the full realization of these transformative treatments. Yet, within these challenges lie opportunities for innovation and collaboration, driving forward the frontiers of cancer research and patient care. We explore the latest advancements, from combination therapies to biomarker discovery, that hold the potential to overcome obstacles and further enhance the therapeutic arsenal against colorectal cancer.

Empowering Patients and Providers:

Empowering patients and healthcare providers with knowledge and resources is paramount to navigating the complexities of immunotherapy and targeted therapies.

From informed decision-making to proactive management of treatment-related side effects, we equip individuals with the tools and insights needed to navigate this evolving landscape with confidence and resilience. By fostering open dialogue, shared decision-making, and comprehensive supportive care, we aim to optimize treatment outcomes and enhance the quality of life for patients confronting colorectal cancer and beyond.

Conclusion:

In the quest to conquer colorectal cancer, immunotherapy and targeted therapies stand as beacons of hope, illuminating the path towards more effective, personalized, and compassionate care. As we continue to unravel the mysteries of cancer biology and therapeutic interventions, let us embark on this journey with unwavering determination and collective resolve. Together, we can forge pioneering paths, transforming the landscape of cancer treatment and ushering in a new era of healing and hope for generations to come.

NUTRITION AND LIFESTYLE

ROLE OF DIIET IN COLORECTAL CANCER PREVENTION AND MANAAGEMENT

In the intricate tapestry of health and well-being, nutrition and lifestyle choices stand as pillars of resilience against the onset and progression of colorectal cancer. As we embark on this exploration, we unveil the profound impact of dietary habits, physical activity, and holistic lifestyle practices in shaping our body's defense mechanisms against this formidable adversary. Within these pages lies a compendium of knowledge, weaving together the latest research, practical insights, and empowering strategies to empower you on your journey towards colorectal cancer prevention and management through nourishing resilience.

Understanding the Link Between Diet and Colorectal Cancer

The foundation of our understanding begins with unraveling the intricate interplay between diet and colorectal cancer risk. From the consumption of processed meats and red meat to the beneficial effects of fiber-rich foods, we delve into the nuances of dietary components that influence the initiation and progression of colorectal cancer. Furthermore, we explore the role of specific nutrients, such as calcium, folate, and antioxidants, in modulating cellular mechanisms implicated in colorectal carcinogenesis. Through a comprehensive analysis of epidemiological studies and clinical trials, we illuminate the pathways through which dietary choices can either mitigate or exacerbate colorectal cancer risk.

Harnessing the Power of Plant-Based Nutrition:

At the heart of colorectal cancer prevention lies the transformative potential of plant-based nutrition. In this section, we embark on a culinary journey through vibrant arrays of fruits, vegetables, whole grains, and legumes, each brimming with phytonutrients and bioactive compounds that confer protection against colorectal cancer. From the Mediterranean diet to Asian-inspired plant-centric cuisine, we uncover the diverse cultural tapestry of dietary patterns renowned for their anti-inflammatory and anti-carcinogenic properties. Moreover, we explore innovative culinary techniques and recipes that empower individuals to embrace the bounty of plant-based nutrition in their daily lives, fostering resilience against colorectal cancer one delicious meal at a time.

Navigating Dietary Challenges and Choices:

In the modern landscape of dietary abundance and convenience, navigating the terrain of optimal nutrition can be fraught with challenges and temptations. In this chapter, we confront the pervasive influence of ultra-processed foods, sugary beverages, and dietary patterns characterized by excessive red and processed meat consumption. Through practical strategies and evidence-based recommendations, we empower individuals to make informed dietary choices that prioritize colorectal health without sacrificing culinary enjoyment or convenience. From mindful eating practices to navigating social and cultural influences, we offer a roadmap for cultivating a nourishing relationship with food that nurtures both the body and the soul.

Embracing Active Living: Exercise as a Catalyst for Colorectal Health

Beyond the realm of nutrition, physical activity emerges as a potent catalyst for colorectal cancer prevention and management. Drawing upon the wealth of scientific evidence, we explore the multifaceted benefits of regular exercise in mitigating colorectal cancer risk through its effects on inflammation, insulin sensitivity, and gut microbiota composition. Whether through brisk walks in nature, invigorating yoga sessions, or heart-pumping strength training routines, we celebrate the diverse spectrum of physical activities that invigorate the body and fortify the spirit against the insidious encroachment of colorectal cancer. Moreover, we delve into the synergistic relationship between exercise and dietary factors, illustrating how their combined effects amplify resilience against colorectal cancer and enhance overall well-being.

Cultivating Holistic Wellness: Mind-Body Practices for Colorectal Health

In the pursuit of colorectal cancer prevention and management, nurturing holistic wellness emerges as an indispensable cornerstone of resilience. In this final chapter, we embark on a transformative journey into the realm of mind-body practices that harmonize the intricate dance between mental, emotional, and physical well-being. From mindfulness meditation to stress-reducing techniques, we unveil the profound impact of cultivating inner peace and resilience in navigating the challenges posed by colorectal cancer. Moreover, we explore the healing power of community support, spirituality, and creative expression as integral components of holistic wellness that foster empowerment and healing in the face of adversity.

Conclusion:

As we draw the curtains on this journey through the labyrinth of nutrition and lifestyle in colorectal cancer prevention and management, we are reminded of the profound resilience that resides within each of us. By harnessing the transformative potential of dietary choices, physical activity, and holistic wellness practices, we not only fortify our bodies against the onslaught of colorectal cancer but also nurture a deeper connection with ourselves and the world around us. Let us embrace this newfound wisdom with gratitude and determination, forging a path towards vibrant health and flourishing well-being, one nourishing choice at a time.

IMPORTANCE OF REGULAR PHYSICAL ACTIVITIES

In today's fast-paced world, where sedentary lifestyles have become increasingly prevalent, the importance of regular physical activity cannot be overstated. As we strive to optimize our health and well-being, incorporating consistent movement into our daily routines emerges as a cornerstone of a balanced lifestyle. In this discourse, we will embark on a journey to explore the profound impact of physical activity on our bodies, minds, and overall quality of life. From unraveling the physiological benefits to delving into the psychological upliftment it offers, we aim to elucidate the transformative power of movement. Join us as we navigate through the intricate interplay between nutrition, lifestyle, and physical activity, illuminating the path towards vitality and longevity.

Body:

1. **The Physiology of Movement:**
   - Understanding the Mechanisms: Delving into the physiological responses triggered by physical activity, including increased heart rate, improved circulation, and enhanced oxygen delivery to tissues.
   - Building Strength and Resilience: Exploring how regular exercise stimulates muscle growth, enhances bone

density, and fortifies the immune system, contributing to overall physical robustness.

- o Metabolic Marvels: Unraveling the metabolic benefits of physical activity, such as improved insulin sensitivity, regulation of blood sugar levels, and mitigation of cardiovascular risk factors.

2. **Beyond the Body: The Psychological Impact of Physical Activity**

- o Elevating Mood and Mental Well-being: Examining the intricate relationship between exercise and mental health, including the release of endorphins, reduction of stress hormones, and alleviation of symptoms associated with anxiety and depression.
- o Enhancing Cognitive Function: Investigating the cognitive benefits of regular physical activity, from improved focus and concentration to the promotion of neuroplasticity and memory retention.

- o Cultivating Resilience: Discussing the role of exercise as a coping mechanism in navigating life's challenges, fostering resilience, and promoting a positive outlook on life.

3. **Integrating Physical Activity into Daily Life:**
   - o Finding Your Rhythm: Exploring diverse forms of physical activity, from structured workouts to spontaneous movement, and identifying activities that resonate with individual preferences and lifestyles.
   - o Overcoming Barriers: Addressing common obstacles to regular physical activity, such as time constraints, lack of motivation, and physical limitations, and offering strategies for overcoming these challenges.
   - o Fostering Accountability: Emphasizing the importance of social support and accountability in maintaining

consistent exercise habits, whether through workout buddies, fitness communities, or digital tracking tools.

4. **Synergy with Nutrition: Maximizing the Benefits**

   o Fueling Performance: Highlighting the symbiotic relationship between nutrition and physical activity, and elucidating the role of macronutrients and micronutrients in supporting optimal exercise performance and recovery.

   o Balancing Energy Intake and Expenditure: Discussing strategies for aligning dietary choices with activity levels to achieve energy balance and promote sustainable weight management.

   o Harnessing the Power of Timing: Exploring the significance of nutrient timing in relation to exercise, from pre-workout fueling to post-exercise refueling, and optimizing nutrient delivery for enhanced performance and recovery.

Conclusion:

As we draw our exploration of the importance of regular physical activity to a close, it becomes abundantly clear that movement is not merely a means to an end but rather a fundamental aspect of human flourishing. From its profound physiological effects on our bodies to its transformative impact on our minds, physical activity emerges as a catalyst for holistic well-being. By embracing a lifestyle that prioritizes regular movement and integrates it seamlessly with nourishing nutrition practices, we embark on a journey towards vitality, resilience, and longevity. Let us heed the call to action, embracing the joy of movement and savoring the myriad benefits it bestows upon us, for in the dance of life, movement is our most faithful companion, guiding us towards a future brimming with health and vitality.

SMOKING CESSATION AND ALCOHOL MODERATION

In the realm of health and well-being, the intricate dance between nutrition, lifestyle choices, and disease prevention is a compelling narrative that continues to unfold. Among the many factors that influence our health outcomes, the relationship between smoking cessation, alcohol moderation, and dietary habits stands out as a pivotal intersection deserving of deeper exploration. In this discourse, we embark on a journey to unravel the intricate web of connections between nutrition, lifestyle choices, and the habits of smoking and alcohol consumption. Through a comprehensive examination of the latest research, practical insights, and empowering strategies, we seek to illuminate the path towards optimal health and wellness.

Smoking cessation represents one of the most significant steps an individual can take towards improving their health and longevity. The detrimental effects of smoking on virtually every organ system of the body are well documented, with an array of serious health consequences ranging from cardiovascular disease and respiratory disorders to various forms of cancer. However, breaking free from the grip of nicotine addiction is a formidable challenge that requires a multifaceted approach encompassing behavioral interventions, pharmacological aids, and supportive environments. Nutrition plays a pivotal role in this journey, offering a powerful toolkit of dietary strategies to support smoking cessation and mitigate withdrawal symptoms. By focusing on nutrient-dense foods rich in antioxidants, vitamins, and minerals, individuals can bolster their immune system, repair cellular damage, and alleviate cravings. Additionally, strategic supplementation with certain nutrients such as vitamin C, magnesium, and omega-3 fatty acids may offer additional support in managing stress and promoting relaxation, thereby reducing the likelihood of relapse.

Moreover, the quest for moderation in alcohol consumption occupies a central place in the pursuit of holistic well-being. While moderate alcohol consumption has been associated with certain health benefits, including a reduced risk of cardiovascular disease, excessive or habitual drinking poses significant health risks and can contribute to a myriad of health problems, including liver disease, neurological disorders, and mental health issues. Nutrition emerges as a key ally in the quest for alcohol moderation, offering a pathway towards greater self-awareness, mindfulness, and balance. By cultivating a diet rich in whole foods, fruits, vegetables, and lean proteins, individuals can fortify their body's natural defenses, enhance liver function, and mitigate the adverse effects of alcohol on metabolic health. Additionally, prioritizing hydration and electrolyte balance through adequate water intake and the consumption of electrolyte-rich foods can help counteract the dehydrating effects of alcohol and promote overall well-being.

In the quest for smoking cessation and alcohol moderation, the power of lifestyle choices cannot be overstated. Cultivating healthy habits such as regular physical activity, stress management techniques, and mindfulness practices can serve as pillars of support, helping individuals navigate the challenges of breaking free from addictive behaviors and establishing sustainable patterns of health-promoting behavior. Furthermore, fostering a supportive social network, seeking professional guidance, and leveraging community resources can provide invaluable assistance on the path towards greater health and wellness.

As we reflect on the intricate interplay between nutrition, lifestyle choices, smoking cessation, and alcohol moderation, we are reminded of the profound capacity of the human body to heal, regenerate, and thrive. By embracing a holistic approach to health that honors the interconnectedness of mind, body, and spirit, we unlock the transformative potential of nutrition and lifestyle choices in fostering vitality, resilience, and longevity. Together, let us embark on this journey of self-discovery and empowerment, forging a path towards a future defined by vibrant health, vitality, and well-being.

COPING STRATEGIES

DEALING WITH EMOTIONS: FEAR, ANXIETY AND DEPRESSION

In the journey of battling against colorectal cancer, emotions play a profound role, often surfacing as fear, anxiety, and depression. These emotions can manifest at various stages, from the moment of diagnosis to undergoing treatment and even into survivorship. Understanding and effectively coping with these emotional challenges is essential for maintaining overall well-being and quality of life. In this comprehensive exploration, we delve into the depths of fear, anxiety, and depression in the context of colorectal cancer, unveiling unique coping strategies to navigate these emotional waters with resilience and courage.

Understanding Fear, Anxiety, and Depression

Fear, anxiety, and depression are natural responses to the diagnosis and treatment of colorectal cancer. The fear of the unknown, anxiety about treatment outcomes, and overwhelming sense of loss and uncertainty can weigh heavily on individuals facing this disease. Fear may stem from concerns about mortality, changes in bodily functions, or the impact of treatment on daily life. Anxiety often arises from the anticipation of pain, discomfort, or potential complications associated with treatment. Depression, characterized by feelings of sadness, hopelessness, and disinterest, may emerge as individuals grapple with the challenges of living with cancer.

The Impact of Fear, Anxiety, and Depression

The emotional toll of colorectal cancer can have significant consequences for both physical and mental well-being. Persistent fear, anxiety, and depression may lead to sleep disturbances, appetite changes, fatigue, and decreased motivation to participate in treatment or self-care activities. Moreover, these emotional struggles can strain relationships with loved ones, diminish the ability to cope with stress, and contribute to a sense of isolation and loneliness.

Coping Strategies: Navigating the Emotional Terrain

Despite the overwhelming nature of fear, anxiety, and depression, there are myriad coping strategies that individuals can employ to navigate these emotional challenges and cultivate resilience in the face of adversity.

1. **Education and Knowledge Empowerment**: Understanding the disease, its treatment options, and potential outcomes can alleviate some of the fear and anxiety associated with the unknown. Seeking reliable information from healthcare providers, support groups, and reputable sources can empower individuals to make informed decisions and regain a sense of control over their circumstances.
2. **Mindfulness and Relaxation Techniques**: Practicing mindfulness, meditation, deep breathing exercises, and progressive muscle relaxation can help individuals manage anxiety and promote a sense of calm amidst the storm. Engaging in these relaxation

techniques regularly can reduce physiological stress responses and enhance emotional well-being.

3. **Expressive Writing and Journaling**: Writing about thoughts, feelings, and experiences related to colorectal cancer can serve as a therapeutic outlet for processing emotions and gaining clarity. Keeping a journal allows individuals to express themselves freely, track patterns in their emotional state, and identify coping strategies that resonate with them.

4. **Seeking Support and Connection**: Connecting with others who understand the challenges of living with colorectal cancer can provide invaluable support and validation. Joining support groups, participating in online forums, or attending counseling sessions can foster a sense of belonging, reduce feelings of isolation, and offer practical advice for coping with emotional distress.

5. **Maintaining a Healthy Lifestyle**: Prioritizing self-care activities such as regular exercise, nutritious eating, adequate sleep, and social

engagement can bolster emotional resilience and enhance overall well-being. Engaging in activities that bring joy and fulfillment, whether it's spending time with loved ones, pursuing hobbies, or enjoying nature, can provide a welcome distraction from cancer-related stressors.

6. **Professional Support and Therapy**: Seeking professional help from therapists, counselors, or psychologists trained in oncology can offer individuals coping strategies tailored to their unique emotional needs. Cognitive-behavioral therapy (CBT), mindfulness-based stress reduction (MBSR), and other evidence-based interventions can equip individuals with practical skills for managing fear, anxiety, and depression effectively.

Conclusion:

Fear, anxiety, and depression are formidable adversaries in the battle against colorectal cancer, but they need not dictate the course of one's journey. By embracing resilience, cultivating self-compassion, and implementing coping strategies tailored to individual needs, individuals can navigate the emotional terrain of cancer with courage and grace. Don't forget, you are not alone in this fight. Reach out for support, draw strength from within, and dare to hope in the face of uncertainty. Together, we can transcend fear, overcome anxiety, and reclaim joy in the journey towards healing and wholeness.

BUILDING A SUPPORT NETWORK

In the journey through the labyrinth of colorectal cancer, one of the most profound and pivotal aspects is the creation of a robust support network. It is within this network that individuals find solace, strength, and resilience to navigate the challenges presented by this formidable disease. In the following discourse, we shall delve deep into the significance of building a support network, explore the various components that comprise it, and elucidate the invaluable role it plays in coping strategies for those affected by colorectal cancer.

The diagnosis of colorectal cancer often initiates a whirlwind of emotions - fear, uncertainty, and anxiety cloud the mind, casting shadows over the path forward. In such turbulent times, the importance of a support network cannot be overstated. It serves as a beacon of hope, illuminating the way through the darkest of days. Whether it be family, friends, healthcare professionals, or fellow survivors, each member of the support network contributes to the tapestry of comfort and encouragement, providing a sense of belonging and understanding that is indispensable in times of adversity.

Central to the construction of a support network is the cultivation of open and honest communication. The exchange of thoughts, feelings, and experiences fosters a sense of camaraderie and solidarity, eradicating feelings of isolation and fostering a sense of unity. Through shared stories and shared struggles, individuals find common ground, forging bonds that transcend the boundaries of illness and infirmity.

Furthermore, a support network serves as a repository of practical assistance and tangible aid. From transportation to medical appointments to assistance with household chores and meal preparation, the collective efforts of the support network alleviate the burdens of daily life, allowing individuals to focus on their journey towards healing and recovery.

Moreover, the support network serves as a source of invaluable guidance and wisdom. Within its folds lie individuals who have walked the path before, who have faced the same trials and tribulations and emerged stronger and wiser. Their insights and experiences offer invaluable perspective, serving as beacons of inspiration and empowerment for those traversing the arduous terrain of colorectal cancer.

In addition to the interpersonal support provided by the network, it is imperative to acknowledge the role of community resources and support groups in bolstering coping strategies. These forums serve as safe havens for individuals to share their stories, express their fears, and seek solace in the company of others who understand their struggles intimately. Through group discussions, educational sessions, and wellness activities, support groups foster a sense of community and belonging, empowering individuals to reclaim agency over their lives and destinies.

Furthermore, the advent of modern technology has expanded the horizons of support networks, transcending geographical barriers and facilitating connections across vast distances. Online support groups, forums, and social media platforms provide virtual spaces for individuals to connect, share resources, and seek guidance from the comfort of their own homes. In an era defined by digital interconnectedness, these platforms serve as lifelines for those who may be physically isolated or unable to access traditional forms of support.

In conclusion, the construction of a support network is an indispensable pillar in the edifice of coping strategies for individuals affected by colorectal cancer. It is within the embrace of this network that individuals find solace, strength, and resilience to weather the storm of adversity. Through open communication, practical assistance, shared experiences, and community resources, the support network serves as a beacon of hope, guiding individuals on their journey towards healing, empowerment, and ultimately, triumph over colorectal cancer.

INTEGRATIVE THERAPIES: MINDFULNESS, YOGA, AND MEDITATION

In the battle against colorectal cancer, coping strategies extend beyond traditional medical treatments. Embracing integrative therapies such as mindfulness, yoga, and meditation offers a holistic approach to healing, nurturing not only the body but also the mind and spirit. This unique note explores the profound impact of these practices on individuals facing colorectal cancer, delving into their therapeutic benefits, practical applications, and transformative potential.

Understanding Integrative Therapies:

Integrative therapies encompass a diverse range of practices that complement conventional medical treatments. Mindfulness, rooted in the cultivation of present-moment awareness, encourages individuals to observe their thoughts, emotions, and bodily sensations without judgment. Yoga combines physical postures, breathwork, and meditation to promote flexibility, strength, and inner harmony. Meditation, in its various forms, facilitates mental clarity, emotional resilience, and spiritual connection. Together, these modalities offer a multifaceted approach to coping with the challenges of colorectal cancer.

The Healing Power of Mindfulness:

Mindfulness serves as a powerful tool for navigating the emotional turbulence that often accompanies a colorectal cancer diagnosis. By fostering a non-reactive awareness of internal experiences, individuals can cultivate resilience in the face of fear, anxiety, and uncertainty. Mindfulness practices such as mindful breathing, body scans, and loving-kindness meditation provide refuge amidst adversity, offering moments of peace and tranquility amid the storm.

Embracing Yoga as a Path to Wellness:

Yoga transcends its physical manifestations to become a transformative journey of self-discovery and healing. Through the practice of asanas (postures) and pranayama (breathwork), individuals with colorectal cancer can enhance their physical vitality and resilience. Yoga nidra, or "yogic sleep," offers profound relaxation and rejuvenation, soothing the nervous system and promoting restorative rest. Beyond its physical benefits, yoga fosters a sense of inner balance and acceptance, empowering individuals to navigate their cancer journey with grace and equanimity.

The Transformative Power of Meditation:

Meditation serves as a sanctuary for the mind, offering refuge from the relentless chatter of thoughts and worries. Whether through mindfulness meditation, loving-kindness practice, or guided imagery, individuals can cultivate a deep sense of inner peace and acceptance. Meditation also facilitates emotional processing and healing, allowing individuals to navigate the complex terrain of grief, anger, and sadness with compassion and self-awareness. By fostering a connection to the present moment and the inherent wisdom within, meditation becomes a potent ally in the journey towards healing and wholeness.

Practical Applications and Considerations:

Integrating mindfulness, yoga, and meditation into the cancer care journey requires careful consideration and adaptation to individual needs and preferences. Healthcare providers play a vital role in guiding patients towards suitable practices and ensuring their safety and efficacy. Mindfulness-based stress reduction (MBSR) programs, yoga classes tailored to cancer survivors, and guided meditation resources offer accessible avenues for individuals to explore these modalities in a supportive environment. Moreover, cultivating a community of fellow practitioners can provide invaluable support and encouragement along the path to healing.

Conclusion:

In the face of colorectal cancer, integrative coping strategies offer a beacon of hope and resilience. By embracing mindfulness, yoga, and meditation, individuals can harness the healing power of mind-body-spirit integration, fostering inner peace, strength, and vitality amidst adversity. As we navigate the twists and turns of the cancer journey, let us cultivate compassion, courage, and presence, drawing upon the transformative potential within each breath and each moment. Together, we can forge a path towards healing, wholeness, and profound well-being in the face of colorectal cancer.

PREVENTION AND EARLY DETECTION

LIFESTYLE CHANGES TO REDUCE RISK

In the realm of healthcare, prevention is often heralded as the most powerful weapon against disease. When it comes to colorectal cancer, the fourth most common cancer worldwide, the significance of preventive measures cannot be overstated. While genetic predisposition certainly plays a role, emerging evidence underscores the profound impact of lifestyle choices in shaping an individual's risk profile for colorectal cancer. This note aims to illuminate the pivotal role of lifestyle changes in mitigating this risk, offering insights into actionable strategies that can empower individuals to take charge of their health and well-being.

Understanding Colorectal Cancer Risk Factors

Before delving into the specifics of lifestyle modifications, it is imperative to grasp the multifaceted nature of colorectal cancer risk factors. While age, family history, and genetic mutations contribute significantly to susceptibility, modifiable lifestyle factors exert a considerable influence on disease development. Sedentary lifestyles, diets high in processed meats and low in fiber, excessive alcohol consumption, smoking, and obesity have all been implicated as key determinants of colorectal cancer risk. By targeting these modifiable risk factors through proactive lifestyle changes, individuals can significantly reduce their likelihood of developing this malignancy.

Dietary Interventions: Embracing a Colorectal-Friendly Diet

Central to colorectal cancer prevention is the adoption of a diet rich in protective nutrients and devoid of harmful components. Emphasizing the consumption of fruits, vegetables, whole grains, and legumes provides a plethora of health benefits, including enhanced fiber intake, which promotes bowel regularity and mitigates carcinogenic effects. Conversely, limiting the intake of red and processed meats, which have been linked to an increased risk of colorectal cancer, is crucial. Furthermore, minimizing the consumption of sugary beverages and highly processed foods can help maintain a healthy weight and reduce inflammation, thereby further lowering cancer risk.

Physical Activity: Moving Towards Optimal Health

In an era characterized by sedentary lifestyles and desk-bound occupations, physical inactivity has emerged as a pervasive public health concern. However, evidence suggests that regular physical activity confers substantial protection against colorectal cancer. Engaging in moderate-to-vigorous exercise for at least 150 minutes per week has been associated with a notable reduction in colorectal cancer risk. Mechanisms underlying this protective effect include improvements in insulin sensitivity, immune function, and bowel transit time. Encouraging individuals to incorporate physical activity into their daily routines fosters not only colorectal cancer prevention but also enhances overall health and well-being.

Weight Management: Striking for a Healthy Balance

Obesity, characterized by an excess accumulation of body fat, represents a significant risk factor for colorectal cancer. Elevated levels of adipose tissue are thought to promote chronic inflammation, insulin resistance, and altered hormonal signaling, all of which contribute to carcinogenesis. Therefore, achieving and maintaining a healthy body weight is paramount to reducing colorectal cancer risk. Implementing strategies such as portion control, mindful eating, and regular physical activity can facilitate weight management and promote metabolic health, thus lowering the likelihood of cancer development.

Alcohol Moderation and Tobacco Cessation: Breaking Harmful Habits

The detrimental effects of excessive alcohol consumption and tobacco use on colorectal cancer risk are well documented. Alcohol, even in moderate amounts, has been shown to increase the risk of colorectal cancer through various mechanisms, including acetaldehyde toxicity and oxidative stress.

Likewise, tobacco smoke contains numerous carcinogens that can initiate and promote colorectal tumorigenesis. Encouraging individuals to moderate their alcohol intake and quit smoking not only reduces their risk of colorectal cancer but also confers myriad health benefits, including cardiovascular protection and improved respiratory function.

Conclusion: Empowering Change for a Healthier Future

In conclusion, the journey towards colorectal cancer prevention begins with a steadfast commitment to embracing lifestyle changes that promote optimal health. By adopting a colorectal-friendly diet, prioritizing regular physical activity, maintaining a healthy body weight, moderating alcohol consumption, and quitting smoking, individuals can significantly reduce their risk of developing this malignancy. However, effecting lasting behavioral change requires more than mere knowledge; it demands support, motivation, and a collective effort to cultivate a culture of wellness. As we navigate the complexities of modern living, let us seize the opportunity to empower ourselves and others to pave the path to prevention, ensuring a healthier future for generations to come.

SCREENING GUIDELINES FOR DIFFERENT AGE GROUPS

Screening Guidelines for Young Adults (Under 50)

Traditionally, colorectal cancer screening has primarily targeted individuals aged 50 and above, as they are considered to be at higher risk. However, recent trends indicate a concerning rise in colorectal cancer incidence among younger adults. Consequently, there is growing recognition of the importance of early screening in this demographic.

For individuals under 50, especially those with a family history of colorectal cancer or other predisposing factors such as inflammatory bowel disease, screening may be recommended at an earlier age. Genetic testing may also be considered to identify hereditary colorectal cancer syndromes, guiding personalized screening approaches.

In addition to traditional screening methods like colonoscopy, alternative modalities such as stool-based tests, virtual colonoscopy, and flexible sigmoidoscopy may be explored for their feasibility and efficacy in this younger age group. Close collaboration between healthcare providers and young adults is crucial to raising awareness and promoting proactive screening practices.

Screening Guidelines for Adults (Ages 50-75)

For individuals aged 50 to 75, regular colorectal cancer screening is strongly recommended by major medical organizations. Colonoscopy remains the gold standard due to its ability to detect and remove precancerous polyps, thus preventing the development of colorectal cancer.

Other screening options include fecal occult blood tests (FOBT), fecal immunochemical tests (FIT), and stool DNA tests, which offer non-invasive alternatives for those averse to colonoscopy or with contraindications for invasive procedures. While these tests are less sensitive than colonoscopy, they provide valuable opportunities for early detection and can be conducted in the comfort of one's home.

The frequency of screening may vary based on individual risk factors, previous screening results, and personal preferences. Shared decision-making between patients and healthcare providers is essential to tailoring screening recommendations to each individual's unique circumstances.

Screening Guidelines for Older Adults (Over 75)

In older adults over the age of 75, the decision to undergo colorectal cancer screening becomes more nuanced, balancing potential benefits with the risks associated with invasive procedures. While age alone should not preclude screening, consideration should be given to life expectancy, overall health status, and individual preferences.

For healthy older adults with a life expectancy of more than 10 years, continuing regular screening may be beneficial in detecting and preventing colorectal cancer. However, for those with significant comorbidities or limited life expectancy, the emphasis may shift towards quality of life and symptom management rather than cancer detection.

Shared decision-making remains paramount in this population, allowing individuals to weigh the potential benefits and risks of screening in the context of their overall health and personal values. Regular discussions with healthcare providers can help older adults make informed choices aligned with their individual circumstances.

Conclusion

In the realm of colorectal cancer prevention and early detection, screening guidelines serve as invaluable tools for guiding clinical practice and promoting public health initiatives. By tailoring screening recommendations to different age groups, healthcare providers can optimize the efficacy of screening efforts while minimizing potential harm. However, it is essential to recognize that screening guidelines are not one-size-fits-all and should be individualized based on risk factors, preferences, and clinical judgment. Through ongoing research, education, and advocacy, we can continue to refine screening strategies and improve outcomes for individuals at risk of colorectal cancer across all stages of life.

UNDERSTANDING FAMILY HISTORY AND GENETIC TESTING

Family history serves as a cornerstone in identifying individuals at increased risk of developing CRC. Research indicates that individuals with a first-degree relative (parent, sibling, or child) diagnosed with CRC are at significantly higher risk themselves. Furthermore, the age at which the relative was diagnosed and the number of affected relatives can further influence risk the assessment. By comprehensively assessing family history, healthcare providers can stratify individuals into different risk categories, allowing for tailored screening recommendations and preventive interventions.

Genetic Basis of Colorectal Cancer:

A deeper understanding of the genetic basis of CRC has revolutionized risk assessment and management strategies. Hereditary CRC syndromes, such as Lynch syndrome and familial adenomatous polyposis (FAP), are caused by specific gene mutations that significantly increase the risk of developing CRC at a young age. Additionally, numerous low-penetrance genetic variants have been identified through genome-wide association studies, contributing to the overall genetic risk profile of an individual. Genetic testing plays a pivotal role in identifying these high-risk individuals, enabling targeted surveillance and preventive measures.

The Role of Genetic Testing:

Genetic testing has emerged as a powerful tool in personalized medicine, allowing for the identification of individuals predisposed to hereditary CRC syndromes and inherited genetic variants. Advancements in genetic testing technologies, such as next-generation sequencing, have made testing more accessible and cost-effective. Pre-test counseling is essential to ensure informed decision-making regarding genetic testing, including discussing the potential implications of test results on medical management and family members.

Implications of Genetic Testing Results:

Interpreting genetic testing results requires a nuanced understanding of the implications for individuals and their families. Positive test results confirm the presence of a pathogenic mutation, warranting intensified surveillance, risk-reducing interventions, and genetic counseling for family members. Negative results provide reassurance but do not eliminate the need for regular screening, as other genetic and environmental factors may contribute to CRC risk. Variants of uncertain significance (VUS) pose challenges in interpretation, requiring ongoing research and collaboration to elucidate their clinical significance.

Integration into Clinical Practice:

Incorporating family history assessment and genetic testing into routine clinical practice represents a paradigm shift in CRC prevention and early detection. Multidisciplinary collaboration between healthcare providers, genetic counselors, and genetic testing laboratories is essential to ensuring the seamless integration of genetic testing into CRC screening programs. Decision support tools and educational resources can aid healthcare providers in effectively communicating the benefits, limitations, and implications of genetic testing to patients.

Conclusion:

In conclusion, understanding family history and genetic testing is integral to a comprehensive approach to CRC prevention and early detection. By harnessing the power of genetic information, healthcare providers can identify individuals at increased risk, implement personalized screening protocols, and initiate preventive measures to reduce the burden of CRC. Moving forward, ongoing research, education, and advocacy efforts are essential to optimize the utilization of genetic testing in clinical practice and improve patient outcomes in the fight against CRC.

LIVING WITH COLORECTAL CANCER

MANAGING TREATMENT SIDE EFFECTS

Living with colorectal cancer presents a multitude of challenges, not least of which are the various treatment side effects that can significantly impact daily life. In this comprehensive exploration, we delve into the realm of managing these side effects, empowering individuals to navigate their journey with resilience and grace. From understanding the physical and emotional toll of treatment to implementing practical strategies for mitigating side effects, this note serves as a beacon of guidance and support for those facing colorectal cancer.

Understanding Treatment Side Effects:

The journey of cancer treatment often brings with it a host of side effects, ranging from physical discomfort to emotional distress. Chemotherapy, radiation therapy, and surgery can each contribute to a unique set of challenges, including nausea, fatigue, hair loss, and changes in bowel habits. It is crucial for individuals to recognize and understand these potential side effects, as awareness is the first step towards effective management.

Physical Side Effects and Strategies for Relief:

Managing physical side effects requires a multifaceted approach that addresses both the symptoms themselves and their underlying causes. For instance, nausea and vomiting can often be alleviated through anti-nausea medications, dietary modifications, and relaxation techniques. Similarly, fatigue may be mitigated by incorporating regular exercise, maintaining a balanced diet, and prioritizing restorative sleep. By adopting proactive measures and seeking support from healthcare professionals, individuals can enhance their quality of life despite the challenges posed by treatment side effects.

Emotional Impact and Coping Mechanisms:

In addition to physical discomfort, living with colorectal cancer can take a significant toll on one's emotional well-being. Feelings of anxiety, fear, and depression are common responses to the uncertainty and upheaval that accompany a cancer diagnosis. It is essential for individuals to prioritize self-care and seek emotional support from loved ones, support groups, or mental health professionals. Engaging in activities that bring joy and fulfillment, such as hobbies, creative pursuits, or spending time with loved ones, can also serve as valuable coping mechanisms during difficult times.

Nutrition and Lifestyle Considerations:

Maintaining a healthy lifestyle is paramount for individuals living with colorectal cancer, particularly when it comes to managing treatment side effects. A balanced diet rich in nutrient-dense foods can help support overall health and alleviate certain symptoms, such as nausea, constipation, or diarrhea. Likewise, staying hydrated, engaging in regular physical activity, and practicing stress-reduction techniques can contribute to improved well-being and resilience throughout the treatment journey.

Communication with Healthcare Providers:

Effective communication with healthcare providers is essential for addressing treatment side effects and optimizing care. Individuals are encouraged to openly discuss their symptoms, concerns, and preferences with their medical team, as this allows for tailored interventions and adjustments to treatment plans as needed. Healthcare providers can offer valuable guidance, support, and resources to help individuals navigate the challenges of living with colorectal cancer and manage treatment side effects effectively.

Supportive Care Services and Resources:

In addition to medical treatment, individuals living with colorectal cancer can benefit from accessing a range of supportive care services and resources. These may include palliative care, pain management, nutritional counseling, and psychosocial support services. Support groups, online communities, and patient advocacy organizations also offer valuable opportunities for connection, education, and peer support. By tapping into these resources, individuals can find strength, solace, and solidarity in their journey with colorectal cancer.

Conclusion:

 Living with colorectal cancer is a journey marked by both adversity and resilience. While the challenges of managing treatment side effects may seem daunting, individuals have the capacity to adapt, thrive, and find meaning amidst the uncertainty. By embracing a holistic approach to care that addresses physical, emotional, and lifestyle considerations, individuals can cultivate resilience and reclaim a sense of agency in their cancer journey. Together, we stand united in our commitment to supporting and empowering those living with colorectal cancer every step of the way.

COMMUNICATING WITH HEALTHCARE PROVIDERS

Communication between patients and healthcare providers is a two-way street that involves sharing information, asking questions, expressing concerns, and collaborating on treatment decisions. Effective communication fosters trust, promotes shared decision-making, and enhances the overall quality of care.

The Importance of Open Dialogue:

Open and honest communication is essential for building a strong and collaborative relationship between patients and healthcare providers. Patients should feel comfortable discussing their symptoms, treatment preferences, and any concerns they may have. Similarly, healthcare providers should actively listen to patients, validate their experiences, and provide clear and accurate information.

Navigating Treatment Options:

Living with colorectal cancer often involves making complex treatment decisions that can have a significant impact on quality of life. Effective communication with healthcare providers is essential for understanding the various treatment options available, weighing the potential benefits and risks, and making informed decisions that align with the patient's goals and values.

Managing Treatment Side Effects:

Many treatments for colorectal cancer, such as chemotherapy, radiation therapy, and surgery, can cause side effects that may affect patients' physical and emotional well-being. Open communication with healthcare providers is key for identifying and managing these side effects, ensuring that patients receive the support and resources they need to cope with treatment-related challenges.

Addressing Emotional Needs:

Living with colorectal cancer can evoke a wide range of emotions, including fear, anxiety, sadness, and uncertainty. It is important for patients to feel comfortable discussing their emotional concerns with their healthcare providers, who can offer empathy, support, and access to mental health resources as needed.

Navigating the Healthcare System:

The healthcare system can be complex and overwhelming, especially for patients facing a cancer diagnosis. Effective communication with healthcare providers can help patients navigate the healthcare system more efficiently, access necessary services and support, and advocate for their needs throughout the treatment process.

Practical Tips for Effective Communication:

- Prepare questions and concerns ahead of appointments to ensure that all important topics are addressed.
- Bring a trusted friend or family member to appointments for support and assistance in remembering information.
- Take notes during appointments to help you remember important details and instructions.

- Be honest and open about symptoms, treatment side effects, and emotional concerns.
- Seek clarification if any information or instructions are unclear.
- Follow up with healthcare providers as needed to address ongoing concerns or changes in health status.

In conclusion, effective communication with healthcare providers is essential for patients living with colorectal cancer. By fostering open dialogue, patients can actively participate in their care, make informed treatment decisions, and receive the support they need to navigate the challenges of living with cancer. Remember, you are not alone on this journey; your healthcare team is here to support you every step of the way.

ADVOCATING FOR YOURSELVES: TIPS FOR NAVIGATING THE HEALTHCARE SYSTEM

Living with colorectal cancer presents numerous challenges, both physical and emotional. From the moment of diagnosis, navigating the complexities of the healthcare system becomes essential for ensuring the best possible care and outcomes. In this comprehensive guide, we will explore the vital role of self-advocacy in managing colorectal cancer and provide practical tips for navigating the healthcare system with confidence and empowerment.

Understanding Your Diagnosis

The journey begins with understanding your diagnosis. Upon receiving the news of colorectal cancer, it's natural to feel overwhelmed and uncertain about what lies ahead. However, taking the time to educate yourself about the disease can empower you to make informed decisions about your care. Familiarize yourself with the specifics of your diagnosis, including the stage of cancer, treatment options, and potential side effects. Don't hesitate to ask your healthcare team questions and seek clarification on any aspects of your diagnosis that may be unclear.

Building a Support Network

Living with colorectal cancer can feel isolating, but you are not alone. Building a strong support network of family, friends, and healthcare professionals is essential for navigating the challenges ahead. Lean on your loved ones for emotional support and practical assistance, and consider joining a support group to connect with others who are facing similar experiences. Remember that seeking support is a sign of strength, not weakness, and allow yourself to lean on others during difficult times.

Communicating Effectively with Your Healthcare Team

Effective communication with your healthcare team is crucial for ensuring that your needs are met and that you receive the best possible care. Be proactive in expressing your concerns, preferences, and goals for treatment. Keep a list of questions and topics to discuss during appointments, and don't hesitate to advocate for yourself if you feel that your concerns are not being addressed. Remember that you are an active participant in your care, and your input is valuable.

Navigating Treatment Options

Colorectal cancer treatment often involves a combination of surgery, chemotherapy, radiation therapy, and targeted therapies. Understanding your treatment options and their potential benefits and risks is essential for making informed decisions about your care. Take the time to research different treatment modalities, and discuss your options with your healthcare team to determine the best approach for your individual needs. Consider seeking a second opinion if you have any doubts or uncertainties about your treatment plan.

Managing Treatment Side Effects

Treatment for colorectal cancer can cause a range of side effects, including fatigue, nausea, hair loss, and changes in bowel habits. Learning how to manage these side effects effectively can significantly improve your quality of life during treatment. Work closely with your healthcare team to develop a plan for managing side effects, and don't hesitate to ask for help if you need it. Incorporating complementary therapies such as acupuncture, massage, and yoga can also help alleviate symptoms and promote overall well-being.

Advocating for Your Rights

As a patient with colorectal cancer, you have certain rights and protections under the law. Familiarize yourself with your rights as a patient, including the right to informed consent, privacy, and access to your medical records. If you encounter any barriers or challenges in accessing care or obtaining necessary treatments, don't hesitate to speak up and advocate for yourself. You have the right to receive high-quality, compassionate care, and it's essential to assert your rights to ensure that your needs are met.

Seeking Emotional Support

Living with colorectal cancer can take a toll on your emotional well-being, and it's essential to prioritize self-care and seek support when needed. Don't hesitate to reach out to a therapist, counselor, or mental health professional if you're struggling to cope with the emotional challenges of cancer. Engaging in activities that bring you joy and relaxation, such as spending time with loved ones, practicing mindfulness, or pursuing hobbies, can also help alleviate stress and promote emotional well-being.

Taking Charge of Your Health

Living with colorectal cancer requires taking an active role in managing your health and advocating for yourself throughout the treatment process. Stay informed about your diagnosis and treatment plan, communicate openly with your healthcare team, and seek support from loved ones and fellow patients. Remember that you are not defined by your cancer diagnosis, and with the right support and resources, you can navigate this journey with strength, resilience, and empowerment.

SUPPORT AND RESOURCES

SUPPORT GROUPS AND ONLINE COMMUNITIES

In the journey of battling colorectal cancer, one of the most profound sources of strength and solace lies in the embrace of support groups and online communities. Beyond the realm of medical treatments and therapies, these interconnected networks offer a sanctuary of understanding, empathy, and shared experiences. Within these spaces, individuals affected by colorectal cancer find companionship, guidance, and a sense of belonging that transcends the boundaries of geography and circumstance. In this discourse, we shall explore the transformative impact of support groups and online communities, celebrating their role as pillars of support and beacons of hope in the fight against colorectal cancer.

The Importance of Support Groups:

Support groups serve as nurturing environments where individuals grappling with colorectal cancer can find refuge amidst the storm. Whether in-person or virtual, these gatherings foster a sense of camaraderie among participants, providing a platform for open dialogue and mutual support. Here, individuals share their stories, fears, and triumphs, finding validation in the shared experiences of others facing similar challenges. Through the exchange of knowledge and empathy, support groups empower participants to navigate the complexities of their diagnosis with resilience and grace.

Benefits of Support Groups:

The benefits of support groups extend far beyond emotional comfort, encompassing a myriad of tangible advantages for participants. Studies have shown that engagement in support groups correlates with improved psychological well-being, reduced feelings of isolation, and enhanced coping mechanisms in individuals affected by colorectal cancer. Moreover, support groups serve as valuable sources of practical information, offering insights into treatment options, symptom management strategies, and resources for navigating the healthcare system. By fostering a sense of community and solidarity, these groups instill hope and optimism in the hearts of participants, reinforcing their resilience in the face of adversity.

The Evolution of Online Communities:

In the digital age, the landscape of support for colorectal cancer has expanded exponentially through the emergence of online communities. These virtual forums transcend the limitations of physical proximity, connecting individuals from diverse backgrounds and geographic locations. Through platforms such as social media groups, online forums, and dedicated websites, individuals affected by colorectal cancer find a global network of support at their fingertips. Here, they can seek advice, share resources, and forge meaningful connections with others on similar journeys, irrespective of time zones or boundaries.

The Impact of Online Communities:

The impact of online communities on the colorectal cancer community is profound and multifaceted. These digital spaces serve as hubs of information dissemination, providing access to a wealth of resources, research updates, and expert insights on the latest advancements in treatment and care. Moreover, online communities offer a platform for advocacy and awareness-raising, amplifying the voices of survivors, caregivers, and healthcare professionals in the global discourse on colorectal cancer. By harnessing the power of technology, these communities foster a sense of empowerment and agency among participants, enabling them to take an active role in their own healthcare journey.

Navigating Challenges and Harnessing Strengths:

While support groups and online communities offer invaluable support, they are not without their challenges. From navigating misinformation to managing conflicts within group dynamics, participants may encounter obstacles along the way. However, by fostering a culture of respect, empathy, and inclusivity, these communities can overcome adversity and emerge stronger together. Through open communication, active listening, and a commitment to mutual support, participants can harness the collective strength of their community to overcome obstacles and navigate the complexities of their colorectal cancer journey with resilience and grace.

Conclusion:

In the tapestry of the colorectal cancer journey, support groups and online communities are the threads that bind us together in unity and solidarity. Through shared experiences, mutual support, and unwavering empathy, these interconnected networks offer a lifeline of hope and healing to individuals affected by colorectal cancer. As we continue to navigate the challenges of diagnosis, treatment, and survivorship, let us embrace the transformative power of community, standing shoulder to shoulder in the fight against colorectal cancer. Together, we are stronger. Together, we are unstoppable.

FINANCIAL ASSISTANCE PROGRAM

Facing a diagnosis of colorectal cancer can be overwhelming, not only emotionally and physically but also financially. The financial burden of medical expenses, treatments, and supportive care can often seem insurmountable. However, amidst the challenges, there exists a network of support and resources aimed at alleviating the financial strain on patients and their families. In this comprehensive guide, we will explore the various financial assistance programs available to individuals affected by colorectal cancer. From insurance coverage to government aid and nonprofit organizations, we will navigate the landscape of financial support, empowering patients to access the assistance they need to focus on their health and well-being.

Understanding the Financial Impact of Colorectal Cancer:

Before delving into the available financial assistance programs, it is crucial to understand the significant financial implications of colorectal cancer. From diagnostic tests and treatments to medications and supportive care services, the costs associated with managing this disease can quickly accumulate. Additionally, many patients may face challenges such as loss of income due to treatment-related side effects or the inability to work. As a result, financial distress can exacerbate the already stressful experience of coping with a cancer diagnosis.

Navigating Financial Assistance Programs:

1. **Health Insurance Coverage:**
   - Understanding your health insurance policy is the first step in accessing financial assistance for colorectal cancer treatment. Patients should familiarize themselves with their coverage details, including deductibles, copayments, and out-of-pocket maximums. Additionally, understanding which medical services and treatments are covered under their plan can

help patients anticipate and plan for potential expenses.

2. **Government Assistance Programs:**
   - Various government programs offer financial assistance to individuals with cancer. Medicare and Medicaid are two primary sources of healthcare coverage for eligible patients. Additionally, the Social Security Administration provides disability benefits for individuals who are unable to work due to their medical condition. Patients can explore these programs to determine their eligibility and access the support they need.

3. **Nonprofit Organizations and Foundations:**
   - Numerous nonprofit organizations and foundations specialize in providing financial assistance to cancer patients. These organizations may offer grants to help cover medical expenses, transportation costs, and other financial needs. Additionally, some nonprofits

provide assistance with housing, utilities, and other essential expenses. Patients can research and reach out to these organizations for support tailored to their specific needs.

4. **Pharmaceutical Assistance Programs:**
   - Pharmaceutical companies often offer assistance programs to help patients access expensive medications at reduced or no cost. These programs, known as patient assistance programs or drug discount programs, may be available for prescription drugs used in the treatment of colorectal cancer. Patients can inquire with their healthcare providers or directly with pharmaceutical companies to explore available options.

5. **Cancer Centers and Hospitals:**
   - Many cancer centers and hospitals have financial assistance programs in place to support patients facing financial hardship. These programs may

offer sliding-scale fees, discounts, or payment plans to help patients manage their medical bills. Additionally, patient navigators or social workers can provide guidance and assistance in accessing financial resources.

Conclusion:

Navigating the financial aspects of colorectal cancer can be challenging, but it is not insurmountable. By understanding the available support and resources, patients can alleviate some of the financial burden associated with their diagnosis and focus on their healing journey. Whether through health insurance coverage, government assistance programs, nonprofit organizations, or pharmaceutical assistance programs, there are avenues for patients to access the financial assistance they need. It is essential for patients to advocate for themselves, seek guidance from healthcare professionals, and explore all available options to ensure they receive the support they deserve. Together, we can empower colorectal cancer patients to navigate the complexities of their financial journey and focus on what truly matters – their health and well-being.

CONCLUSION

As we reach the culmination of our journey through the intricate world of colorectal cancer, it is imperative to reflect on the insights gained, the challenges faced, and the paths ahead. Throughout this comprehensive exploration, we have traversed the landscape of this disease, from its inception to its management, shedding light on its complexities and empowering both patients and caregivers alike.

Our odyssey began with an in-depth understanding of the fundamentals of colorectal cancer, illuminating the intricate biology and mechanisms underlying its development. We delved into the anatomy of the colon and rectum, unraveling the intricate interplay of genetic mutations, environmental factors, and lifestyle choices that contribute to the initiation and progression of this disease. By comprehending the origins of colorectal cancer, we lay the groundwork for informed decision-making and proactive prevention strategies.

Moreover, our exploration extended beyond mere knowledge acquisition, delving into the realm of early detection and diagnosis. We emphasized the paramount importance of screening and surveillance in identifying colorectal cancer at its nascent stages, thereby enabling timely intervention and an improved prognosis. Through discussions of various screening modalities and diagnostic techniques, we empowered individuals to advocate for their health and seek timely medical attention when warranted.

Furthermore, our journey traversed the landscape of colorectal cancer treatment, exploring the myriad therapeutic modalities available to patients. From surgical resection to adjuvant chemotherapy and targeted therapies, we navigated the intricacies of treatment decision-making, emphasizing the importance of individualized care and multidisciplinary collaboration. Through discussions of treatment efficacy, potential side effects, and supportive care measures, we sought to alleviate the burdens borne by patients and caregivers alike, fostering resilience and hope in the face of adversity.

Yet, our exploration extended beyond the confines of medical intervention, encompassing the broader domains of nutrition, lifestyle modification, and psychosocial support. We underscored the pivotal role of diet and exercise in mitigating disease risk and enhancing treatment outcomes, advocating for holistic approaches to wellness that encompass mind, body, and spirit. Moreover, we delved into the realm of emotional well-being, offering strategies for coping with fear, anxiety, and uncertainty while fostering resilience and empowerment in the face of adversity.

As we bid farewell to this odyssey through the realms of colorectal cancer, it is essential to acknowledge that our journey is far from over. While we have traversed vast terrain and acquired invaluable insights, there remain uncharted territories and unanswered questions yet to be explored. Thus, as we navigate the path forward, let us do so with a spirit of curiosity, resilience, and collaboration, recognizing that our collective efforts hold the potential to transform the landscape of colorectal cancer care.

In conclusion, our journey through the realms of colorectal cancer has been one of discovery, resilience, and hope. From the intricacies of disease biology to the complexities of treatment decision-making, we have ventured forth with courage and determination, guided by a shared commitment to improving outcomes and enhancing quality of life. As we stand on the precipice of possibility, let us embrace the challenges and opportunities that lie ahead, forging a path towards a future where colorectal cancer is but a distant memory and the promise of wellness beckons for all.

Together, let us embark on this journey with renewed vigor and determination, united in our pursuit of a world free from the scourge of colorectal cancer.